D0844296

Podiatric Medicine and Surgery
A Monograph Series

Managing Editor:
Morton D. Fielding, D.P.M.

Volume I:	Surgical Treatment of Hallux-Abducto Valgus
Volume II:	Surgical Treatment of the Intractable Plantar Keratoma
Volume III:	Skin Tumors of the Foot: Diagnosis and Treatment
Volume IV:	Podiatric Sports Medicine
Volume V:	Soft Somatic Tumors of the Foot
Volume VI:	Surgical Treatment of Digital Deformities

Podiatric Sports Medicine

by

Steven I. Subotnick, D.P.M., M.S.

Associate Professor of Biomechanics and Surgery,
California College of Podiatric Medicine

Executive secretary, American Academy of Podiatric Sports
Medicine Member, American Medical Joggers Association

Member, American College of Sports Medicine

Diplomate, National Board of Podiatric Surgery

Fellow, American Academy Podiatric Sports Medicine

illustrator

Stanley G. Newell, D.P.M., A.C.F.S.

Clinical Instructor, Department of Ambulatory and
Community Medicine, California College of Podiatric Medicine

Consultant in Sports Medicine, University of Washington

Director, First Year Surgical Residency Program
Waldo General Hospital, Seattle

**FUTURA
PUBLISHING COMPANY
1975**

The three following appendices are reprinted by permission of the Journal of the American Podiatry Association:

The Biomechanical Basis of Skiing reprinted from *JAPA,* Volume 64:1, January 1974.

Compartment Syndromes in the Lower Extremities reprinted from *JAPA,* Volume 65:4, April 1975.

The Short Leg Syndrome reprinted from *JAPA,* Volume 66, 1976.

Second printing—1979

Published by
Futura Publishing Company, Inc.
295 Main Street
Mount Kisco, New York 10549

L.C. #: 74-82021
ISBN #: 0-87993-044-6

Dedication

To my wife Janice and my children Mark, Ali, and Kari

Foreword

The following chapters are somewhat informal in structure and make no pretense to be other than a guide for health practitioners in sports medicine.

It has been my intention to relate my experiences in sports medicine to the reader as a practicing podiatrist as well as an active long-distance runner and skier.

As with most of my self-serving projects these past few years, my wife and family have born the brunt. I lovingly thank my wife Janice, son Mark, and daughters Ali and Kari for allowing me my indulgences.

Apart from my family I gratefully thank Dr. Stan Newell, podiatrist from Seattle, Washington, for his fine illustrations used in this book as well as Dr. George Sheehan and Joe Henderson for their friendship and constant encouragements. I thank Ms. Cathy Florendo for the massive job of typing and retyping that she did. And I thank most sincerely those tremendous patients of mine who not only insisted upon my entrance into sports medicine but also nurtured me into my major pastime of long-distance running. The rewards of treating an athlete successfully are equaled only by those of becoming an athlete oneself.

CONTENTS

Foreword

Chapter 1: The Athlete and the Sports Medicine Podiatrist 1

Chapter 2: History and Physical for the Athlete 5

Chapter 3: The Biomechanics of Running 13

Chapter 4: Normal Functioning of the Foot in Walking Race Walking and Running 21

Chapter 5: Structural and Functional Lower Extremity. Abnormalities Which Produce Abnormal Foot Function 33

Chapter 6: Overuse Syndrome of the Foot and Leg 47

Chapter 7: Foot Types and Injury Predilections 57

Chapter 8: Shin Splint Syndrome of the Lower Extremity 79

Chapter 9: Dynamic Muscle Imbalance (Runner's Equinus) 83

Chapter 10: Orthotic Foot Control for the Athlete— The Importance of Resupination 87

Chapter 11: The Abuses of Orthotics in Sports Medicine 93

Chapter 12: The Field Treatment of Athletic Overuse Injuries (First Aid) 97

Chapter 13: The Use of Tape for Prevention and Treatment of Lower Extremity Athletic Injuries 105

Chapter 14: Chondromalacia of the Knee and Related Conditions 115

Chapter 15: Soft Tissue Disorders of the Foot and Leg 125

Chapter 16: Bony Abnormalities of the Foot Which Affect the Athlete 139

Chapter 17: Surgical Correction of the Intractable Soft Tissue and Bony Abnormalities of the Athlete's Foot 149

Appendix 1: Compartment Syndromes in the Lower Extremities 181

Appendix 2: The Short Leg Syndrome 189

Appendix 3: The Biomechanical Basis of Skiing 195

Chapter 1

The Athlete and the Sports Medicine Podiatrist

INTRODUCTION

The athletes that the sports medicine podiatrist see fall into four basic categories. The first group consists of the junior high and high school students. The second group consists of the college athletes. The third group consists of the white collar workers who are health and recreation enthusiasts and are training for their respective sports. The fourth group consists of the professional athletes who are dependent upon their performance for their livelihood. Each of these groups has its own special considerations which warrant the attention of the doctor. All groups have one basic characteristic in common. Injury is defined in their terms as the inability to train or compete. They rarely present with the more common symptoms of the generally less active public. The underlying pathology may be the same but the increased stress of athletes usually results in more serious soft tissue and bony damage.

THE ATHLETE

The junior high and high school students are prone to injury which could result in permanent damage. Paramount are those injuries to the epiphyseal areas of the long bones. In addition, soft tissue injuries not treated properly can result in permanent damage to muscle-tendon units or can lead to unstable and lax joints. Despite pressure from an occasional over zealous parent or coach, it is usually advisable to protect the younger athletes at all times from the hazards of competing or participating with soft tissue or bony injuries. These young athletes have many useful, productive, enjoyable seasons of athletic endeavors ahead of them if they are taught to train properly and if they respect the first warning signs of injuries. The younger athletes may outgrow some of their structural imbalances, but greatly benefit from functional, protective, orthotics while they are growing. They respond very well to a biomechanically sound approach to their injuries. Occasionally, the younger patients will appear to have nothing organically or structurally wrong. In these cases, the parents should be interviewed. Often times it will be realized that the young athletes are not happy with or well suited to the sport chosen for them by their well-meaning, yet over zealous parents. This has occurred several times to me over the past years in my practice. Finding a sport more suited to the younger athletes' temperament and body type and skills, while playing down the importance of competition and the importance of participation, appeared to have worked well in these patients.

Although college athletes may be dependent on their performance to maintain athletic schorlarships, it is still the doctor's responsibility to protect these athletes from damaging themselves in an irreversible manner. Certain steps should be taken to protect the athletes while allowing for competitions. These athletes, especially, must be encouraged to use proper training and conditioning methods. In addition, they should be given protective devices including foot orthotics and strappings when indicated.

The third group of athletes consists of the white-collar college graduates who wish to stay in shape. These athletes are extremely dedicated to their athletic endeavor which is an intricate part of their life. They will consider anything to avoid quitting respective sports. The sports more commonly undertaken by the white-collar workers include jogging, long-distance running, bike riding, tennis, golf and skiing. To suggest that these athletes should stop their involvement in their selected sport, will insure the doctor a loss of the patient. These patients will go from doctor to doctor until they can find one that will try to somehow find a way to allow them to continue with their athletic endeavor while not further injuring themselves. Although these athletes can usually be treated successfully by outlining conditioning and training programs, and utilizing functional orthotics, occasionally there are those who are so ill-suited for their sport, that suggestions to participate in another sport are in order. This group of athletes traditionally is wary of all forms of medicine (especially surgery) and responds best to your sincerity in approaching their problems.

The fourth group of athletes is the most difficult to treat. These are the professional athletes who must compete at any cost. They need instant treatment and success for all problems no matter how severe. They seldom are interested in long-term therapy programs and are often willing to take the consequences of competing with an injury. The doctor must stress the severity of the injury and the long-term consequences of competition without proper rest or treatment. The professional athletes, by and large, through the process of natural selection, are less prone to many of the injuries that affect white-collar athletes. Despite this, they are often injured and even more often are never afforded a biomechanically sound functional approach to their injury.

THE BRINK OF DISASTER

All athletes have one thing in common; the better trained they are the closer they are to being on the brink of disaster. The *brink of disaster* is that state between athletic excellence and athletic disaster. Too much training can lead to injury. The injury might be of any type from a pulled gastrocnemius to a chondromalacia of the patella or a partial rupture of the plantar fascia. Stress is vital for conditioning, but too much stress is detrimental to the athlete's health. Overstress can lead to the symptoms of generalized fatigue and a susceptibility towards contagious diseases such as influenza and colds.

Sports and athletics, by their very nature, are stressful. Training is merely adapting to stressful situations. There must be a balance between necessary stress and overstress. Without this balance the athlete falls into the brink of disaster. This situation is avoided by proper warming up, training, conditioning and warming down. In addition, the use of functional orthotics greatly aid the athlete to overcome the overuse syndrome.

THE PODIATRIST IN SPORTS MEDICINE

Since all athletic endeavors involve some form of walking or running and since this is dependent on proper lower extremity and foot function, it seems logical that the podiatrist should be one of the key physicians dealing with sports medicine problems.

Each sport has its own individual characteristics, but all sports consist of movements on the three body planes. These movements are either transverse plane rotation, sagittal plane acceleration and decelerations, or frontal plane movements. Specifically by biomechanical control of the foot, motion on all these planes can be affected, as well as the athlete's speed, agility and ability to withstand overuse and overstress.

The sports medicine doctor is one who knows the sports of his various athlete patients and can converse with them on their own terms. He knows of their training schedules and conditioning habits and can point out weaknesses in their daily routines. He can correlate overdevelopment of various muscle groups which are peculiar to each sport with the possibility or probablity of injuries. He can advise as to proper flexibility, strength and functional exercises which fit in well with proper training and conditioning routines. The sports medicine doctor serves as a good example if he himself is an athlete. He must believe in the importance of athletics for total mind and body health. Athletes are generally turned off by a doctor who appears to be grossly out of condition and overweight. Although the sports medicine doctor may not have actively participated in many of the sports he is involved with as a doctor, he can become familiar with these sports by going to the games, talking to coaches and analyzing movies of the various motions which take place in these sports. The sports medicine doctor should also be knowledgeable in the different forms of footgear and special equipment available to him. Examples of this are ski boots and bindings, types of tennis and running shoes, jogging and track shoes, hiking boots, and variations in soccer and football shoes.

The sports medicine podiatrist must act as a doctor as well as a counselor and at times even as a coach. The decisions he makes can be heartbreaking for the athlete, parents and coach, but above all, must protect the patient.

Chapter 2

History and Physical for the Athlete

HISTORY OF PRESENT ILLNESS

The chief complaint of the athlete is usually parapharased from the athlete's own words and should, as clearly as possible, pinpoint the actual complaint or complaints. Athletes will often times have one primary complaint and several smaller complaints. Overtraining and overuse is a big contributing factor and it often affects more than one area of the lower extremity.

The injury etiology is either sudden or gradual. Gradual injuries begin as nagging pain during running and end as acute pain even when walking. These types of histories suggest overuse as well as biomechanically faulty structure, as an etiology.

Sudden injury, such as an acute rupture or strain, suggests an explosive injury, possibly related to an improper warm-up or a traumatic incident.

Injuries apparent only after a workout suggest, again, overuse. Injuries occurring after races or competition, as compared to workouts, can be related to changes in distance, pace, or terrain. An example of this is an injury occurring when running on hills after spending much time training on flat terrain.

Some injuries are related to unaccustomed changes in foot gear. An example of this is a transition from training shoes with a high heel to racing spikes with no heel. This places an unaccustomed strain on the tendo Achillis.

Many injuries are related to terrain changes. For example, going from a grass field to an asphalt road or from clay tennis courts to cement courts. Often times shin splints are common when the runner goes from outdoor surfaces to an indoor track. There are different injuries on artificial turf as compared to natural turf.

An injury may be related to progressive abnormal shoe wear. An example of this is increasing wear on the outside aspect of the heel. The more the outer aspect of the heel wears, the more the weight is thrown to the outside. I have had patients whose injury parallels the amount of abnormal wear on the shoe.

CLASSIFICATION OF OVERUSE INJURIES

The athlete generally considers a serious injury as one he cannot run through. Anything less is a mere inconvenience. Therefore, careful questioning will reveal other injuries which may fit a particular pattern. Injuries are termed *first degree* if bothersome and hurt only before and after running activities, but are generally asymptomatic during the actual run. These injuries generally get worse without the proper training and functional control of the lower extremities. These are the types of injuries that are usually ignored until they become more serious and bring the athlete to the doctor's office. They generally progress to the point where activity must be limited and no fast running allowed. Then the runner will only be able to run on the flats and hill running will cause increased pain. The tennis player may limit himself to not rushing to the net. The basketball player may not be able to rebound and the football player may have to eliminate cutting.

The *second degree* injuries are those that are beyond just being bothersome. The athlete has pain before, during, and after activity, although he is able to participate, somewhat, in his chosen sport.

Injuries reach the *third degree* status when no activity is possible in the chosen sport, although alternative sports are still possible. An example of this is a runner who has taken up riding a bike while mending from a running injury or a basketball player who must swim while he is recuperating.

Fourth degree injury status is reached when no activity, even walking, is possible. A first degree injury may very well progress to a fourth degree injury when there is total lack of treatment or concern for the injury.

FURTHER PRESENT ILLNESS CONSIDERATIONS

When ascertaining a history of the present illness, the doctor should also concentrate on three main topics: training, conditioning and functioning.

With *training,* the type of mileage and speed per mile, the duration of activity, and type of terrain are all important. Examples are hills and flat areas. The duration of a type of workout and the frequency of injuries with this workout are important. Past history of similar injuries treated professionally or by the athlete himself should be evaluated.

When considering *conditioning,* it is important to appreciate the type of workout exercises which are carried out both pre and post workout. Is the athlete doing any flexibility or strength exercises? Are weights being used for strength or for repetition? Are any special medications or diets being used connected with the sport? How often is the athlete competing?

In regard to *functioning,* we would want to know if the athlete feels that he is functioning with one leg doing something different than the other leg. Is there repeated injury in one leg compared to the other leg? If the athlete is a jumper, does he have more problems on his takeoff or on his landing foot and leg? If the athlete is a golfer, is there more problem on the back or forward foot? If the athlete is a skier, can he turn only to the right or only to the left without getting injured?

PAST MEDICAL HISTORY

The past medical history is a scanning of the medical, surgical, traumatic and allergic history of the athlete. In the older athletes, the medical history can be significant, especially if this athlete is running or jogging after a previous heart attack or has a history of cardiopulmonary disease. If the athlete is a beginner, in regard to jogging, and has not had a proper medical evaluation prior to his undertaking this activity, it is always advisable to refer him to the family physician or internist for a further medical workup.

A social and familial history are often times useful when faced with a more difficult diagnosis, such as the "pushy parent" syndrome or the very competitive compulsive individual who is prone to overstress.

THE PHYSICAL EXAMINATION

The physical examination of the athlete in our office consists initially of examining that portion centered around the chief complaint. Examples include the ankle, foot, plantar fascia, knee, leg, thigh, or hip. Specific anatomical considerations will be covered in further sections. Following a thorough examination of this anatomical part, the patient then is examined in gait. A thorough gait analysis is useful in directing the podiatrist towards possible causes of injuries. At times it is necessary to observe the athlete actually performing in his athletic endeavor, but this is rarely done on the initial visit. We do, on occasion, have the athlete jog for us in the hallways so that we can compare normal walking to their jogging activities. Following the gait analysis, the athlete is then examined for muscle strength and balance, as well as flexibility. Range-of-motion evaluation and examination are carried out and include motion evaluations of the back, hip, knee, ankle, subtalar and midtarsal joints. The subtalar neutral position is determined as is the neutral position for the midtarsal joints. Neutral stance is compared with compensated stance. Tibial varum and calcaneal valgus are recorded. Talar-navicular relative congruency is evaluated[22,23] (Figure 1). A functional position is ascertained. This position is explained to the athlete as the position for maximum efficiency for his function. This is the position which has the least chance for overuse injury when utilized in functional foot orthotic control.[37] Biomechanical determinations will be further discussed in the following sections. This biomechanical examination is vital to ascertain the functional reasons behind the athlete's particular injury.[38]

Athletes with a possible cardiovascular problem have vital signs evaluated and the heart and lungs are auscultated. Deep tendon reflexes are routinely checked as well as normal sensations. A more involved neurologic examination is called for in cases of nerve entrapment, low back syndrome and sciatica. In these situations, pelvic symmetry as well as limb length is evaluated (see Appendix 3).

The peripheral vascular status is evaluated as a matter of routine.

Following the initial history and physical, attention is then directed towards specific indicated tests.

Special Tests

X-ray examination of the feet and other injured areas of the lower extremity are carried out on the initial visit. When fractures are suspected, a stat reading is obtained. In cases of ankle injury, a stress view may be indicated. Foot X rays are routinely taken in the weight-bearing attitude so that functional interpretations can be made. When indicated, various lab tests are ordered. Certain conditions may require diagnostic nerve blocks (see Chapter 15). This will be discussed in further sections.

FIGURE 1
Morphological Data Chart

STEVEN I. SUBOTNICK, D.P.M., M.S.

MORPHOLOGICAL DATA CHART

LEFT		RIGHT
	SUBTALAR JOINT:	
INVERSION °	SUPINATION	INVERSION °
EVERSION °	PRONATION	EVERSION °
°	TOTAL R.O.M.	°
VARUS ° VALGUS	NEUTR[illegible]	VARUS ° VALGUS
VARUS ° VALGUS	MIDTA[illegible]	VARUS ° VALGUS
	ANKLE JOINT:	
DORSIFLEXION °	RANGE OF DORSIFLEXION } c̄ KNEE EXTENDED	DORSIFLEXION °
DORSIFLEXION °	RANGE OF PLANTARFLEXION } c̄ KNEE EXTENDED	DORSIFLEXION °
DORSIFLEXION °	RANGE OF DORSIFLEXION } c̄ KNEE FLEXED	DORSIFLEXION °
DORSIFLEXION °	RANGE OF PLANTARFLEXION } c̄ KNEE FLEXED	DORSIFLEXION °
	ANKLE TO KNEE:	
INTERNAL ° EXTERNAL	MALLEOLAR TORSION	INTERNAL ° EXTERNAL
INTERNAL ° EXTERNAL	ABNORMAL TRANSVERSE KNEE ROTATION	INTERNAL ° EXTERNAL
	HIP JOINT:	
c̄ HIP FLEXED | c̄ HIP EXTENDED		c̄ HIP FLEXED | c̄ HIP EXTENDED
° | °	RANGE OF INTERNAL ROTATION	° | °
° | °	RANGE OF EXTERNAL ROTATION	° | °
° | °	TOTAL R.O.M.	° | °
° | °	NEUTRAL POSITION	° | °
	GENU DEVIATION:	
VARUM ° | VALGUM ° | RECURVATUM °	I.M. DISTANCE ____ cm.	VARUM ° | VALGUM ° | RECURVATUM °
	STANCE CORRELATION:	
VARUM ° VALGUM	FRONTAL PLANE TIBIA	VARUM ° VALGUM
ADDUCTION • ABDUCTION	ANGLE OF GAIT	ADDUCTION • ABDUCTION
INVERTED ° EVERTED	CALCANEAL STANCE POSITION IN STATIC ANGLE OF GAIT	INVERTED ° EVERTED
INVERTED ° EVERTED	CALCANEAL POSITION TO FLOOR SUBTALAR JOINT NEUTRAL	INVERTED ° EVERTED
PRONATION ° SUPINATION	RESULTANT ABNORMAL SUBTALAR JOINT POSITION	PRONATION ° SUPINATION

SUMMARY: ____

____

DISPOSITION

An initial impression is reached, and the athlete is advised as to the need of altered or improved training, conditioning and functioning. The training and conditioning considerations are outlined on instruction sheets and functional foot control is obtained by using various types of foot orthotics. Specific local treatment to relieve pain is instituted when indicated, as will be explained in further sections. A biomechanical explanation as to etiology and then treatment aimed towards improved function and balanced structure achieves the total patient approach. When local treatment is used, the patient must be warned that this is only temporary and that further follow-up is necessary for total rehabilitation (Figure 2).

Often times I will utilize a temporary soft orthotic in order to evaluate the effects of relatively functional control for the athletic injury. This is fabricated and dispensed on the first visit and may allow for continued training while recovering from an injury. Types of orthotics are discussed in further detail in Chapter 10.

FURTHER CONSULTATION

Further consultation is at times desirable from other medical colleagues. I have utilized the orthopedist, neurologist, neurosurgeon, family physician, internist, pediatrician, physical therapist, and other podiatrists.

SUMMARY

In summary, then, the sports medicine podiatrist must be aware of the individual needs of the various athletes he treats. He must be well-versed in the proper training, condition, and functioning required for each sport. He should seek biomechanical explanations for functional problems. The sports medicine doctor should be well aware of the various forms of athletic foot gear available for each sport with advantages and disadvantages of each. Above all, the doctor must realize the importance of the sport to the athlete, for mental and physical well-being, and accept his role in returning the athlete to activity while preventing further or recurrent injury. The philosophy that the mere absence of disease does not mean physical fitness is paramount in the sports medicine doctor's understanding of the athlete.

FIGURE 2
EXERCISES FOR FEET AND LEGS

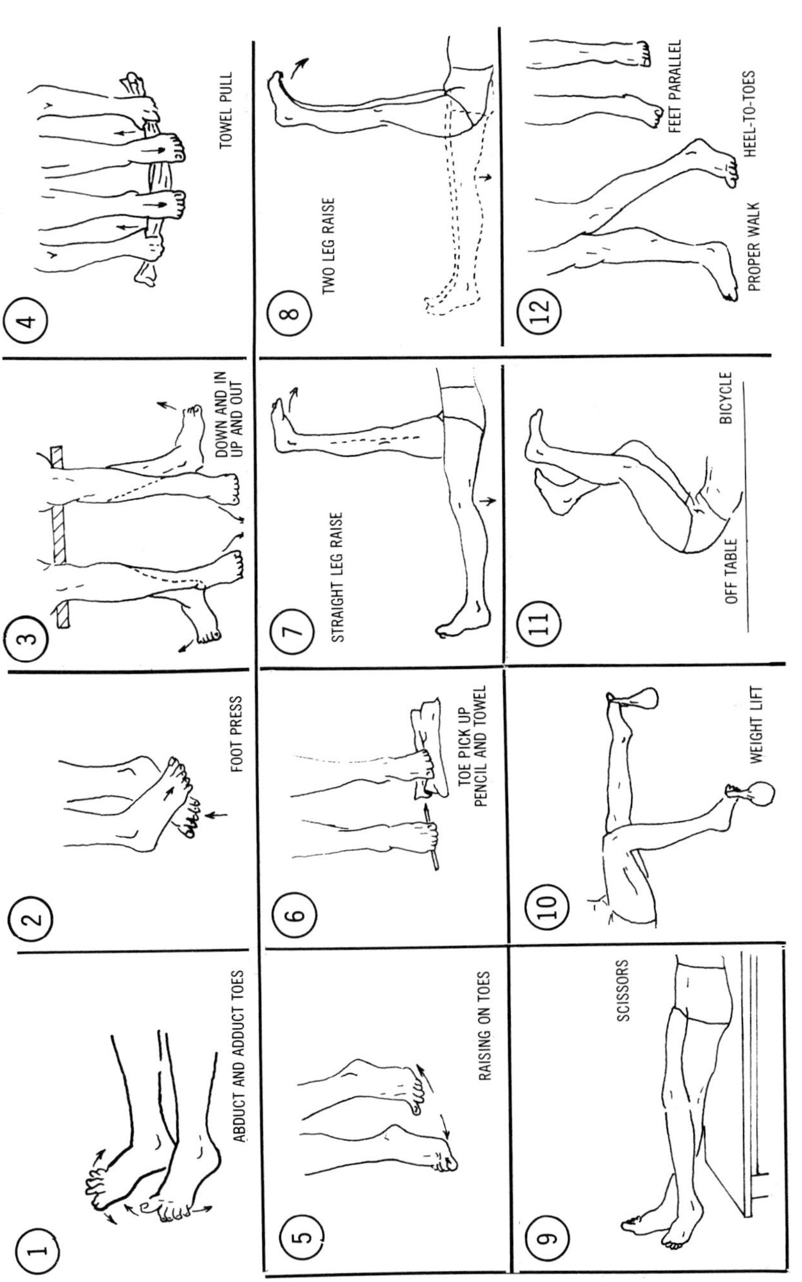

Exercises #1 to #6
Move ankles, feet and toes SLOWLY through these exercises.

Exercises #7 and #8
Raise one leg at a time, lowering slowly. Then raise both legs together and lower slowly.

Exercise #9
Raise legs up 2″ from floor or bed and slowly cross and uncross them.

Exercise #10
With 10 pound weight across foot, elevate alternately the right leg, then the left leg, to 90°.

Exercise #12
When walking, keep feet parallel and finish step on the toes (not on ball of foot).

Chapter 3

The Biomechanics of Running

INTRODUCTION

The human foot is a complex structure which is designed to convert the rotations of the leg and upper extremity into meaningful, translatory forward motion. Normal locomotion places a great deal of stress upon the foot as it accepts the body weight from above and it attempts to adjust to varying changes in the walking surface. Jogging and running produce even greater stresses and, when normal foot function is not present, overuse breakdown at the lower extremity is possible.[1, 3, 5, 25, 29] The normal locking and unlocking of joints is necessary to dampen the stress of normal locomotion and running. A normal range of motion is necessary or else this dampening action will be lost.[23, 37, 38] This further adds to the overuse syndrome which is present with improper biomechanical function. A normal foot is one which, during function, places no undue stress upon itself, or the joints proximal to it; the ankle, knee or hip joint. Normal does not mean average in as much as the average function of the foot for a given population may be abnormal. Abnormal function over a period of time may very well lead to soft tissue and bony deformities of the lower extremity; preventative treatment of abnormal function appears necessary. A knowledge of the biomechanics of running is a prerequisite for attempting to control abnormal foot function in the runner. In as much as running is a part of most athletic endeavors, understanding and correcting abnormal foot functioning during running, allows us to help many athletes.[38, 29]

KINEMATICS OF WALKING

Familiarity with the biomechanics of walking is a prerequisite for an appreciation of the biomechanics of running. Normal walking is comprised of the swing phase (35%) and the stance phase (65%), of a total cycle lasting from heel strike to heel strike (Figure 1). During the swing phase the foot is not in contact with the ground and the lower extremity is internally rotating. During the first 15% to 25% of the stance phase of gait, at which time heel and then foot make contact with the ground, the limb is still internally rotating.[23] The foot, however, cannot internally rotate due to the reactive forces of the contacting surface which prevent this type of motion. Therefore, the foot is dependent upon the subtalar joint, a universal type joint, which allows for internal, transverse plane rotation of the leg to be manifested in the foot by closed kinetic chain pronation. This results in the apparent rolling in of the ankle as the calcaneus everts and is accompanied by concommittant lowering of the medial longitudinal arch of the foot. This combination of first subtalar and then midtarsal joint pronation often times results in an unstable foot. The pronated foot, however, functions as a mobile adaptor on uneven ground surfaces. Subotnick[32] has alluded to the ill effects of the hypermobile foot during the propulsive phase of the gait. Although mobility is desired during the contact phase of gait it is undesireable during the toe-off phase. Pronation, thus, allows for the foot to adapt to heel contact to uneven surfaces. This is a very useful function for such activities as golfing, hiking, running or even walking in the sand. Too much pronation, however, which does not reverse itself, can often cause symptoms of malfunction and overuse.

FIGURE 1
THE GAIT CYCLE IN WALKING

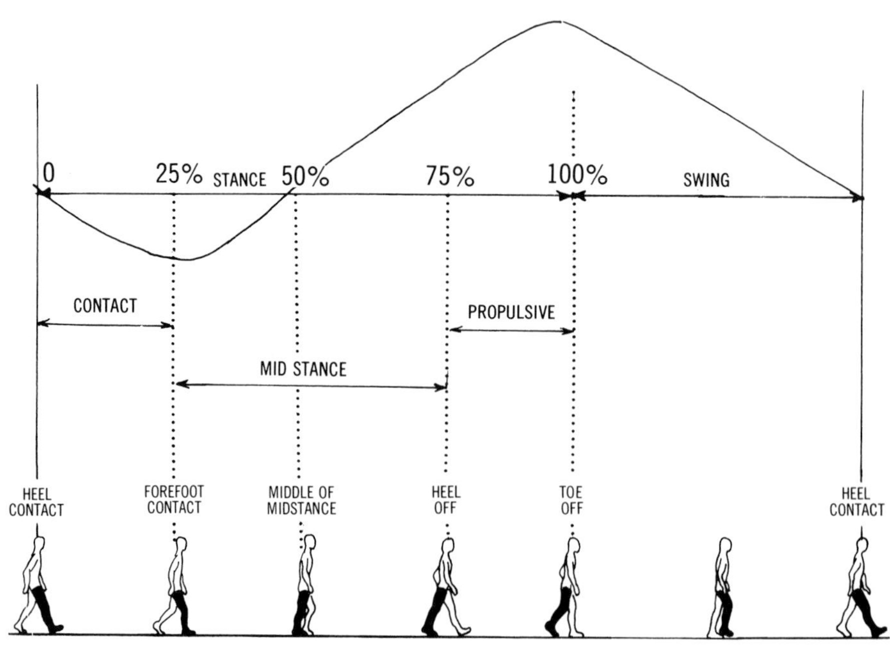

During the midstance of gait the foot becomes more rigid and at toe-off should be a rigid lever as the leg is externally rotated. Thus, we note that from mid-stance to toe-off, the foot supinates as the leg externally rotates. This results in a raising of the medial longitudinal arch. Supination prepares the foot to act as a rigid lever and enables a strong, powerful toe-off to occur. This is necessary for normal ambulation and for forceful propulsion. If abnormal or prolonged pronation occurs at heel strike which does not correct itself in allowing the foot to become a rigid lever, a proper toe-off cannot occur and along with the loss of power in stride, various postural symptoms occur.[32] (See Chapter 4.)

Figure 1 demonstrates the stance phase and swing phase of the normal ambulation foot and we note that the stance phase consists of the foot acting as a mobile adaptor during the first 15% to 25% (the contact portion of gait) and that the leg is internally rotating during this period of time. During the midstance portion of gait, which is the middle 50% of the stance phase, the leg is externally rotating and the foot is moving from the attitude of a mobile adapter to that of a more rigid structure for acceptance of kinetic stress and preparation for toe-off. The foot is thus moving out of pronation and into supination. The remaining 25% of the stance phase of gait comprises toe-off and this occurs when the heel leaves the ground. At this time the first ray is actively being plantarflexed around its independent axis and at the same time the remainder of the foot is actively supinating and becoming a very rigid lever. This stabilizes both the medial and lateral column of the foot and allows for the structures inserting into the great toe to provide for a very powerful toe-off. Hypermobility or lack of resupination results in deformities ranging from sheer callouses underneath metatarsal heads to hallux valgus and hammer toe deformities.[36] In addition, it has been noted that the pronated foot at toe-off has a tendency to adversely effect the ankle, knee and leg and results in many overuse symptoms in the athlete. Neutral orthotic control of the foot is obtainable for normal walking. By relating the kinematics and biomechanics of walking to running, one can gain knowledge as to the importance of neutral control in running. Thus, we must investigate the various types of running and kinematics involved, as previously done with walking.

KINEMATICS OF RUNNING

Running varies from normal ambulation by the fact that there is an intervening air-borne period when neither lower extremity is in contact with the supporting surface. In normal ambulation, one foot is always on the ground. Slocum and James [27] (Figures 2 and 3) have divided running into a support phase which consists of three periods: foot strike, mid-support and take-off. The recovery phase is divided into the periods of follow-through, forward-swing and foot-descent. Foot strike begins when the foot first touches the running surface and continues for a brief moment during which the foot becomes firmly fixed. Mid-support begins once the foot is fixed and continues until the heel begins to rise from the running surface. Take-off begins when the heel begins to rise and continues until the toes leave the running surface.(Figures 2 and 3)[27].

During the recovery phase follow-through begins as the trailing foot leaves the ground and continues until the foot ceases its rearward motion. Forward swing begins with the beginning of forward motion of the foot and terminates when the foot reaches its most forward position. Foot-descent begins after the recovery foot reaches its most forward position, reverses direction and descends toward the running surface in a rearward direction and terminates with foot strike.

A review of the figure illustrating the phases in running from Slocum and James illustrates that the phases for running are similar to those of ambulation and that the contact foot goes through similar motions. This is, of course, dependent upon the speed of running. During the support phase, sprinters have a tendency to stay on the ball of a foot, although the heel may sag towards the running surface during mid-support. Middle-distance runners often contact the running surface on the ball of the foot initially and the heel may momentarily strike the running surface. In longer distance runners, foot strike may be with the heel, or heel and forefoot simultaneously contacting the running surface. Joggers often go through a heel-foot-toe type of gait. During the support phase the foot must first act as a mobile adaptor and then very quickly convert itself into a rigid lever by supinating to allow for a powerful toe-off. At mid-support in running one notes that the tibia is about perpendicular to the running surface and that the foot should be close to a neutral position. Just beyond this mid-support the leg swings forward approximately 10 degrees on the neutral foot [32]. This is analogous to what we see in normal ambulation and suggests to us that lack of flexibility of the posterior muscle groups will lead to overuse symptoms.[38] James pointed out that the foot must be acclerated over a very short distance to the same velocity as that of the body so that at foot strike the foot is moving close to zero velocity in relation to the supporting surface to minimize the horizontal force creating a breaking action on the body's center of gravity.

FIGURE 2

THE GAIT CYCLE IN RUNNING

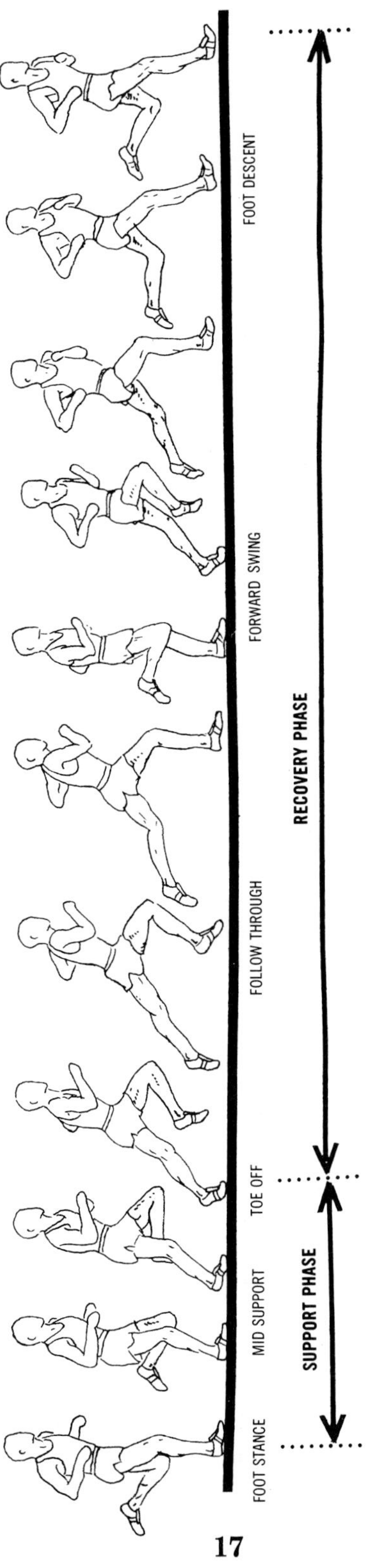

FIGURE 3
BIOMECHANICS OF RUNNING

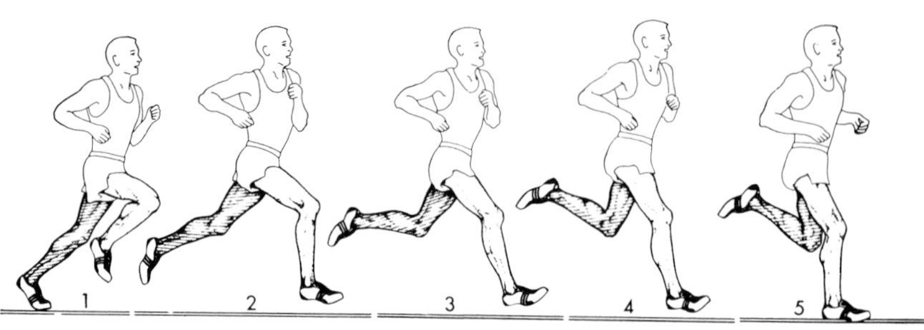

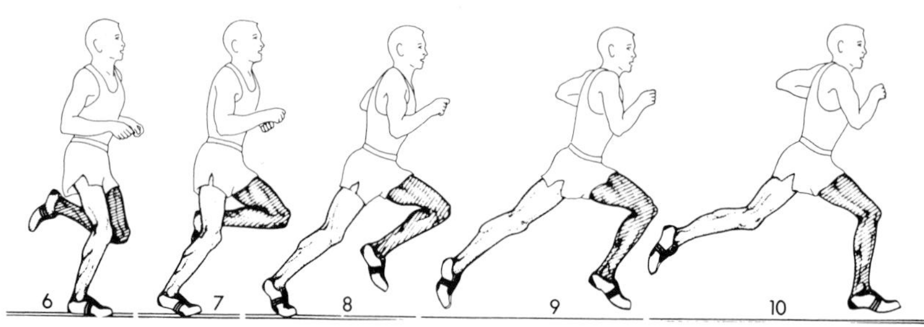

This is not true, however, during changes of velocities such as accelerations, deceleration or change of direction during which time there is considerable horizontal components of force at foot strike. At the instant of foot strike the foot makes contact with the ground initially in a supinated position and as weight is accepted proceeds into pronation until the forefoot is securely fixed to the running surface. The right hip is internally rotating and extending during this period. From this period of initial contact until toe-off, the limb then externally rotates. At toe-off the lower extremity then begins to internally rotate. We, thus, see an analogous situation between running and walking wherein pronation occurs at heel strike and supination occurs throughout the remainder of the period of time that the foot is on the ground to allow the foot to convert from a mobile adaptor to a rigid lever to accept stress and to allow for a powerful thrust at toe-off, or at least a stable hallux.

KINEMATICS - CORRELATIONS BETWEEN WALKING AND RUNNING

A review of slow motion films of sprinters, middle-distance runners and long-distance runners suggests the following: joggers and long-distance runners go through a heel-foot-toe type of gait in which the foot functions are very much the same as encountered in normal ambulation. The heel strike may be quite abrupt and jarring, or may be shortened by a rapid heel strike then with total foot contact. Some joggers and long-distance runners contact the supporting surface initially flat-footed. This "slap-footed" contact may also be jarring, expecially when the foot is pronated (flattened) at contact. Middle-distance runners appear to contact on the ball of their foot and then have their heel sag back to contact the supporting surface, and then go into a ball-of-the-foot and toe-off phase. Sprinters, as was pointed out by James, contact and remain on the ball of their foot.[27] It is further noted that sprinters coming out of starting blocks, have a tendency to abduct and pronate their feet at the beginning of their starts to allow for more secure contact of the foot with the running surface. After this initial take-off phase they begin to point their feet in a more straight ahead pattern and do not pronate as severely. We have been able to correlate prolonged pronation with an abducted angle of gait and suggest that this may result in the situation of lowered efficiency in running. Counter-clockwise track competition allows for supinating forces upon the left foot and pronating forces upon the right foot in the turns.

SUMMARY

A review of the biomechanics of running and correlation with normal ambulation allows one to compare the similarities and differences. We have seen that running may be divided into a support phase and a recovery phase consisting of foot strike, mid-support and take-off roughly corresponding to the contact, mid-stance, and propulsive phase of normal ambulation. It becomes apparent that devices (orthotics) that control a foot in normal ambulation may be modified to also control abnormal motion in running. Further investigation of the kinematics of running, and especially that of the foot function allows us to better provide for proper foot control for athletes.

Chapter 4

Normal Functioning of the Foot in Walking, Race Walking and Running

INTRODUCTION

It is theoretically concluded that given an athlete, with proper and sensible training and conditioning, and a biomechanically sound and normal lower extremity, injury should be kept to a very low level. This, of course, precludes the collision injuries and those severe twisting injuries that take place from very irregular surfaces, such as falling into a chuck hole or wrenching an ankle on loose dirt. It is, therefore, necessary to understand what is normal, what is ideal, and what deviations from the ideal and conditions of normalcy, preclude to injury. A normal foot is one, which during function, places no undue stress upon itself or the other joints proximal to it: the ankle, knee or hip joint. Normal does not mean average, in as much as the average function of the foot for a given population may be biomechanically or structurally abnormal for certain activities.[37,38] The average foot is not suited for standing all day on man-made surfaces, such as cement, although this is a normal activity for many people. The average and normal foot is not suited for long hours of pounding the tennis courts, basketball courts, or long road runs on sidewalks or asphalt. Inasmuch as abnormal function over a period of time very well may lead to soft tissue and bony deformities as well as injuries of the lower extremities, preventative correction of abnormal function appears necessary. Criteria for normalcy shall be presented.

NORMAL FOOT FUNCTION

An understanding of normal foot function in walking is essential before one can understand and correlate this understanding to normalcy and abnormalcy in jogging, running and other forms of athletic movement. This is particularly important because mild to moderate deviations from normal foot functions in walking can produce symptoms far more severe in the athlete than in the nonathlete. Thus, moderate biomechanical deformities of the lower extremities, particularly the foot, can produce severe disabling injuries.

A biomechanically sound lower extremity is one which has the bisection of the calcaneus parallel to the bisection of the lower 1/3 of the leg when both feet are resting on the ground in bipedal stance (Figure 1). This is the same normalcy which should exist at the middle of mid-stance in any one gait cycle.(See Figure 3 in Chapter 3.) In bipedal stance the osseous stability of the foot, due to the biomechanically sound structure, should make it necessary only for mild contractures of the anterior and posterior muscles to maintain balance. The structural stability of the foot in bipedal stance is the basis for support of the foot.[23] This is different during kinetic situations in which cases, the various muscles, tendons, and soft tissue-structures of the foot, must function in such a way to move the foot into positions that will favor stability.[37]

FIGURE 1
THE NORMAL FOOT AND LEG

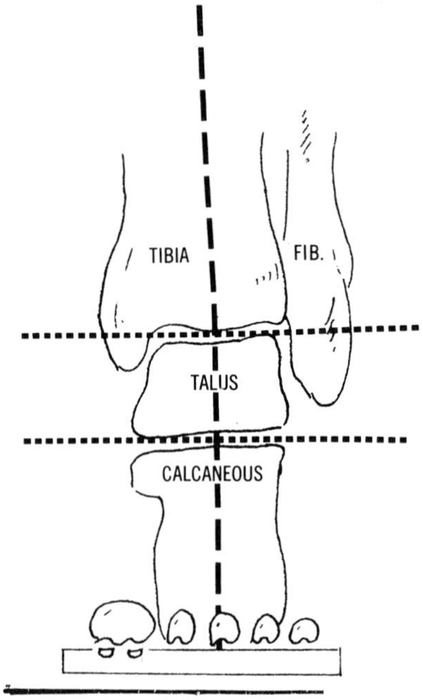

During movement, central programming allows for sequentially proper resupination to occur providing normal structure is present. Proper resupination is the basis for efficiency as well as injury prevention. In bipedal stance, in the biomechanically sound lower extremity, the tibia lower one third is perpendicular to the ground and its bisection is parallel to the posterior surface of the calcaneus (Figure 1). The calcaneus is thus in its neutral position. From this position, the calcaneus can usually move into eversion and inversion (Figure 2). It usually moves into inversion twice as much as it can into eversion. Thus, if a total subtalar joint range of motion which is manifested by the calcaneus inverting and everting, is 30 degrees, this normal subtalar joint would show 10 degrees eversion and 20 degrees inversion. This same biomechanically sound foot would have all of the metatarsal heads resting on the ground with a good longitudinal and transverse metatarsal arch. This is possible by the locking of the midtarsal joint which occurs when the subtalar joint is in its neutral position and the midtarsal joint is maximally pronated. (A maximally pronated midtarsal is one which will not allow for a collapse or pronation of the foot beyond the perpendicular calcaneal position despite the amount of lateral pressure upon the forefoot.) Thus, a maximally pronated midtarsal joint, with a neutral subtalar joint, allows for all metatarsal heads to rest on the ground with osseous stability of the foot (Figure 1).[32, 33]

An athlete is examined in his basic angle of gait, that angle which the foot forms from the line of progression, in bipedal stance. Once can then determine if his feet are close to this biomechanically sound or neutral position, or deviate from it. Deviations from this ideal situation make it difficult for the various muscles, tendons and soft tissue structures of the lower extremity to move the foot into a position that will allow for stability during walking and running. The neutral subtalar joint and maximally pronated, neutral, mid-tarsal joints are essential for the foot to become rigid and allow the muscle tendon units to provide for a powerful thrust at propulsion. Loss of good propulsion means loss of efficiency, a chance for injury, and an increase in the overuse syndrome, which is common to athletes. (See Chapter Six.)

THE GAIT CYCLE

The gait cycle can be divided into two major phases, the swing phase which is 35 percent of the total gait cycle, and the stance phase which is 65 percent of the total cycle. One gait cycle is from heel strike to heel strike (See Figure 3 in Chapter 3).[23]

Swing Phase of Gait

During the swing phase of gait in normal ambulation, the swinging foot and leg are internally rotating. This internal rotation of the thigh and leg takes place for the first 15 to 25 percent of the stance phase of gait, at which time the heel and then the foot meet with the ground. The limb becomes part of a closed kinetic chain reaction at heel contact. The heel must evert with closed kinetic chain pronation and thus the foot becomes a mobile adapter at contact.

FIGURE 2
The Neutral Position of the Subtalar Joint

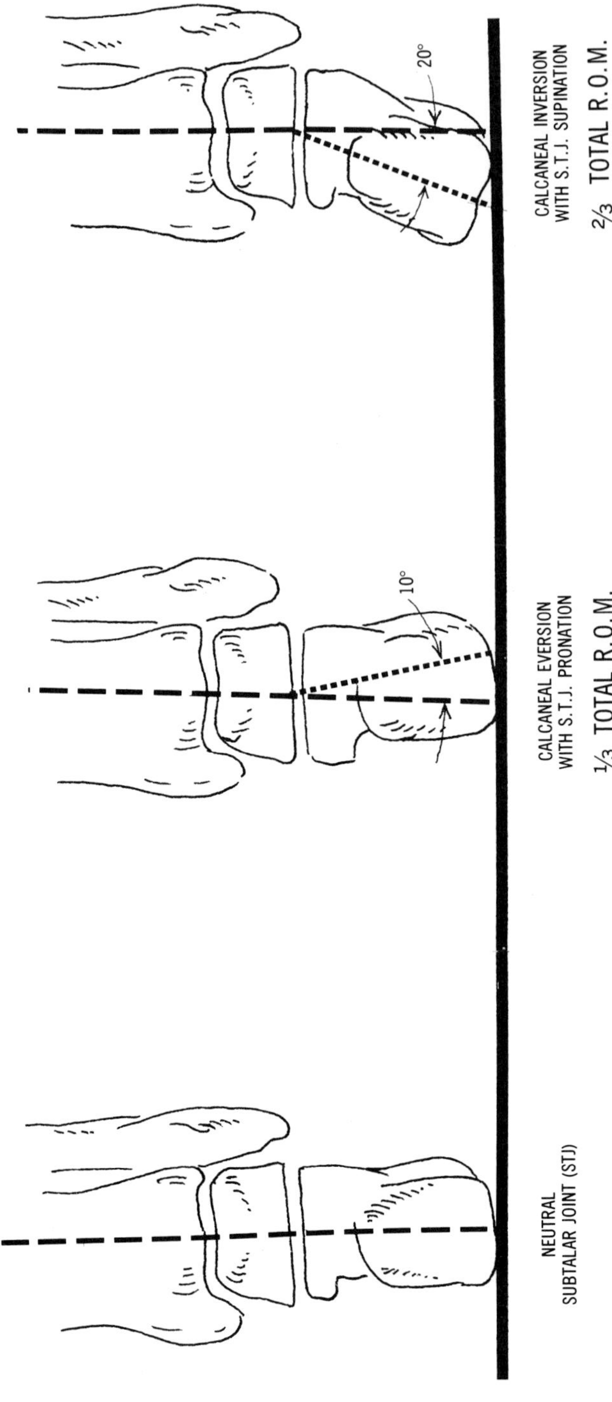

Contact Portion of Stance Phase

Internal rotation of the leg, when the foot is on the ground is synonymous with closed kinetic chain pronation and indicates that the foot is becoming a mobile adapter during the contact portion of the stance phase of gait. This is an unstable foot, but a foot which can accommodate varying surfaces. This contact portion pronation is entirely normal for proper function. Approximately four degrees of contact pronation are necessary for normal function. To stop this normal pronation will increase the jarring effect of contact and can produce various overuse syndromes. As the leg internally rotates at contact with closed kinetic chain pronation, the foot must pronate because it cannot internally rotate due to the reactive forces of the contacting ground which prevent any type of motion other than that which occurs on the frontal plane, i.e., eversion or inversion of the calcaneus (Figure 1). Therefore, the foot is dependent upon the subtalar joint, a universal type of joint, which allows for transverse plane rotation to be absorbed in the foot by either eversion or inversion of the calcaneus. This is, of course, pronation or supination of the subtalar joint.

Subtalar joint pronation unlocks the midtarsal joint and allows the full forefoot to accommodate various changes in terrain. The midtarsal joint has two axes of motion. The primary motion at the oblique axis is dorsiflexion and plantarflexion. On the longitudinal axis the primary motions are inversion and eversion. These various axes can allow for motion independent from each other. Subtalar joint pronation, thus, allows for the foot to adapt at heel contact to uneven surfaces. This is normally a very useful function and essential to those sports taking place on uneven surfaces, i.e., golf, cross country running, and hiking. Contact pronation dampens the shock of heel strike by the locking and unlocking of the joints. Excessive and prolonged pronation, which does not reverse itself, will often times cause symptoms associated with malfunction and overuse. Thus, pronation which lingers on beyond 15 to 25% of the stance phase of gait is abnormal and causes torques in the lower extremities which lead to an overuse syndrome.

Mid-stance Portion of Stance Phase of Gait

Following the contact portion of gait is the mid-stance portion which is characterized by single support in normal walking and is the middle 50% of the stance phase (Figure 3). During this portion the lower extremity transverse plane rotations reverse themselves and the thigh and leg externally rotate.

FIGURE 3
COORDINATED GAIT CYCLES OF BOTH LOWER EXTREMITIES

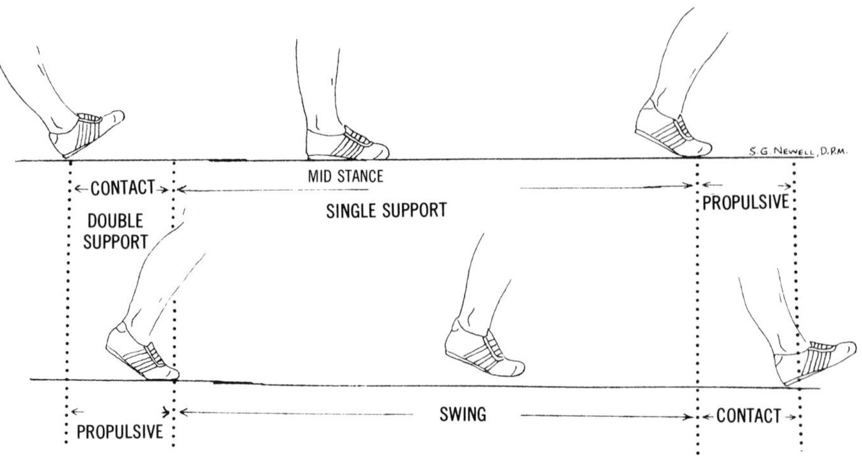

External rotation in a closed kinetic chain is synonymous with supination of the foot. The foot thus moves from a directon of pronation to a direction of supination. It moves from a mobile adapter to a rigid lever as it prepares itself for a stable toe-off. This motion towards rigidity is important to allow for the various tendons of the leg to function around stable bony levers.

Just preceding the middle of mid-stance, the tibia swings over the talar dome about ten degrees (See Figure 2 in Chapter 3). At this instant the foot is neutral and the leg is perpendicular to the ground with the knee almost maximally extended. This is the reasoning for ten degrees of dorsiflexion of the neutral foot being necessary to avoid the compensatory pronation which occurs at the subtalar and midtarsal joints if this forward swing of the leg is impeded by a functional or true equinus. (Figures 1 and 2)[32]

Just following the middle of midstance is heel-off (See Figures 1 and 2 in Chapter 3). The foot is now moving from a neutral to supinated position and the heel inverts from two to four degrees as the arch raises and the foot becomes more of a rigid lever. (Figure 4)[32]

Early heel-off indicates an uncompensated or partially compensated equinus. Prolonged heel-off parallels prolonged abnormal pronation.

Supination of the subtalar joint locks the midtarsal joint so that the stable pully and lever systems are present. Abnormal or prolonged pronation demands internal rotation of the leg when external rotation should be taking place. This causes abnormal torques at the hip, knee and ankle joints as well as within the foot.

FIGURE 4

TRANSVERSE PLANE ROTATIONS OF THE LEG AND ITS EFFECT UPON THE FOOT

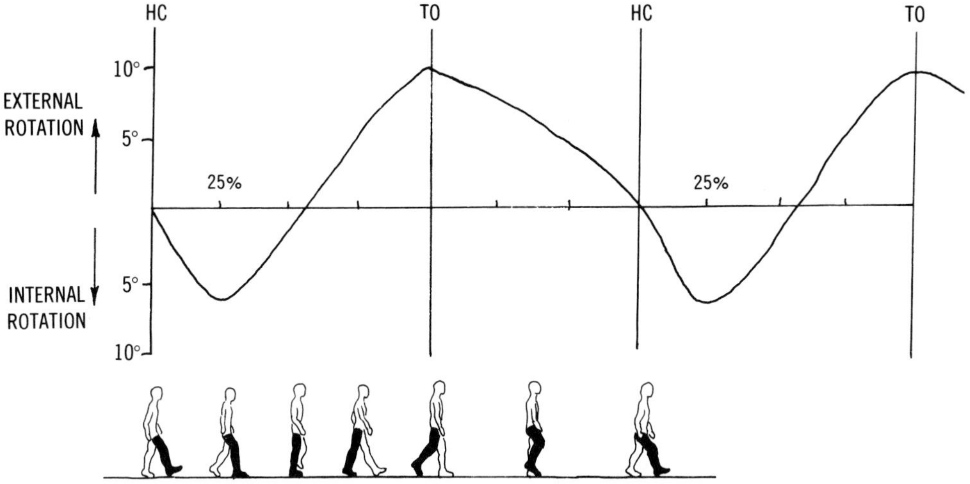

FIGURE 5

PROLONGED PRONATION OF THE FOOT IN THE ATHLETE

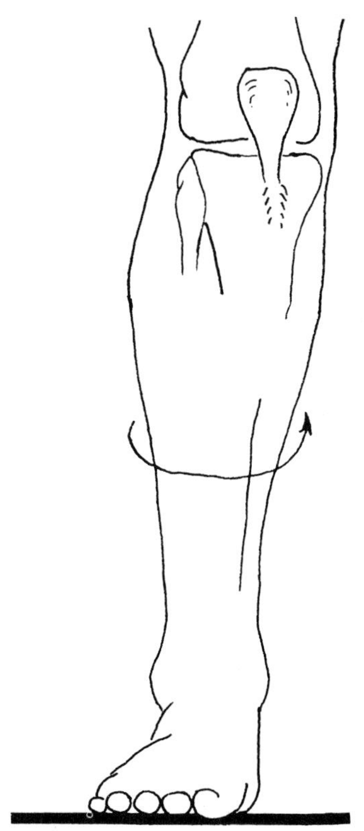

This also precludes a normal stable great toe. The great toe bears the greatest amount of weight at toe-off and without stability toe-off is very inefficient. Thus, prolonged abnormal pronation taking place during mid-stance causes increased overuse syndromes, over fatigue, and a generally less efficient stride and less efficient athletic performace. Prolonged pronation prolongs the onset of resupination and decreases its stabilizing effect at toe-off (Figures 4 and 5).

Stride variations occur with various postural symptoms. Pronation is not bad. It is necessary and useful. Lack of resupination during the mid-stance of gait is bad and leads to a myriad of athletic injuries. Lack of resupination which can be visualized when the athlete is walking, also takes place when the athlete is running.

Propulsive Portion of Gait

The last 25% of the stance phase of gait is the propulsion portion. This is again a bipedal portion with the heel of the opposite leg contacting as toe-off is occurring on the stance foot. The majority of the weight of the foot during the propulsive phase of gait is transferred from the first metatarsal out to the great toe. Prolonged mid-stance pronation produces an apropulsive gait and in effect there is no real propulsive action. Depending upon the extend of abnormal pronation, a foot may resupinate during the swing phase or else remain pronated throughout the swing phase and contact the surface already maximally pronated.

THE NORMAL FOOT IN RACE WALKING (8 MINUTES PER MILE TO 6.5 MINUTES PER MILE)

Race walking is basically a fast form of walking with the knee very close to being fully extended at heel contact. Contact is far back on the heel and then the foot goes through a normal gait pattern. Race walking is much faster than normal walking and as the speed of gait increases, less time is spent with an individual foot on the ground. The swing phase becomes increased and the double support phase becomes minimal. Thus, in race walking, as one heel comes down, toe-off is occurring on the other foot and most of the stance phase of gait is single support. In race walking there is no float phase and either one foot or both feet are on the ground (Figure 6).

FIGURE 6
COMPARISON OF STANCE AND SWING PHASES OF GAIT IN WALKING, RACE-WALKING, JOGGING AND SPRINTING

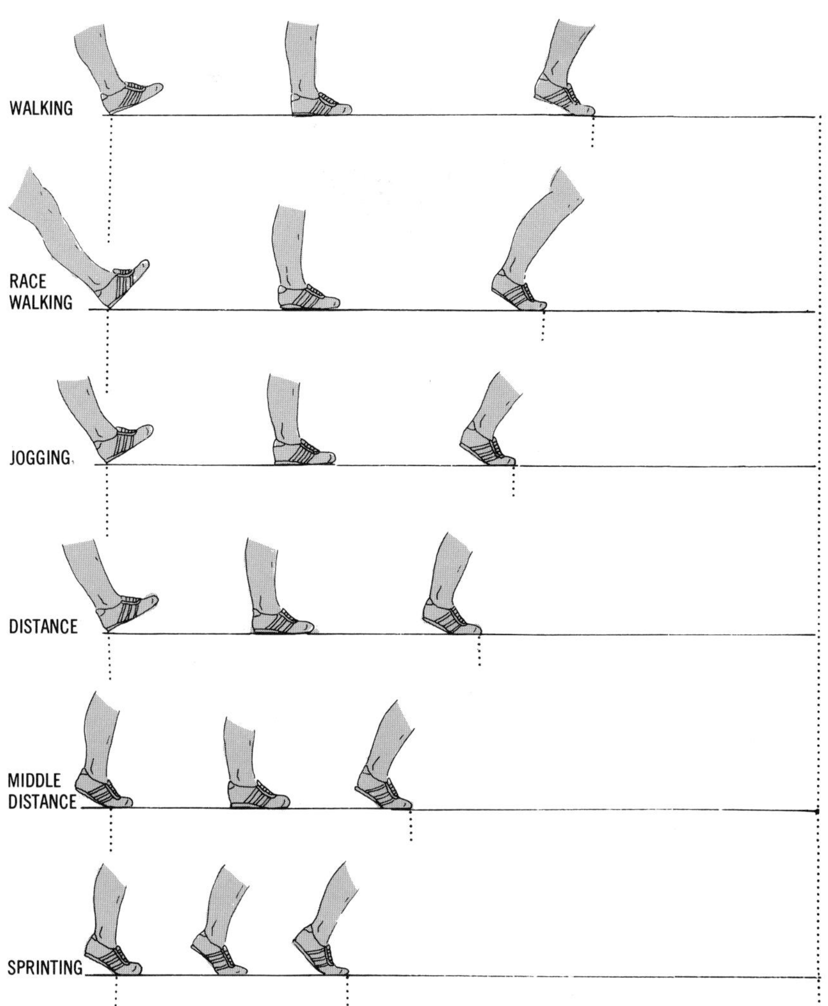

JOGGING (EIGHT PLUS MINUTES PER MILE)

During jogging there is a float phase which takes place. This is a period of no support (Figure 6). In jogging there is either a single support or no support. The swing phase becomes even longer as the stance phase shortens. The stance phase, however, is longer than the swing phase. The foot still goes through the same axis motions as occurs in normal ambulation. There is a contact, a mid-stance and propulsive portion.

In race walking and jogging, at the middle of mid-stance, the normal biomechanical sound foot positioning should be present. This is the neutral foot which should occur during bipedal stance. This is the foot with the subtalar joint in a neutral position and the midtarsal joint maximally pronated and neutral. This is the foot with the bisection of the lower one third of the tibia parallel to the bisection of the posterior surface of the calcaneus (Figure 1). Although with jogging, the contact, mid-stance and propulsive portions of gait are shortened, occurring more rapidly, it is important to realize that the same basic principles and concepts necessary for a biomechanically sound walking pattern apply to a biomechanically sound jogging and running pattern (Figure 4).

LONG-DISTANCE RUNNING (6-26 MILES)

In long-distance running, the swing phase and stance phase approach each other. The stance phase is just a bit longer than the swing phase. A long-distance runner may run anywhere from six to twenty miles a day. The running pace varies from eight minutes to five minutes per mile. With this type of mileage, it is paramount for biomechanically sound function to be taking place in the lower extremities (Figure 3).

DISTANCE RUNNING (1-6 MILES)

In distance running, the swing phase and the stance phase of gait are for equal amounts of time. A distance runner is usually a one to three miler. He will be competing at speeds faster than long-distance runners, but his foot still goes through the basic heel-foot-toe type of gait. (Figure 3)

MIDDLE-DISTANCE RUNNERS (440 YDS.-MILE)

Middle-distance runners have a shorter stance phase than swing phase of gait. During their swing phase of gait they are floating through space. They make contact on the ball of their foot, rock back to their heel and then have a very explosive propulsive phase. The middle-distance runners are the half-milers and milers. Even with these runners the middle of mid-stance should allow for a neutral foot positioning (Figure 3).

SPRINTERS (50 - 440 YD. DASHERS)

The sprinters are the 100,110, and 440 yard men. They usually remain on the balls of their feet for most of the race. Some 440 yard men contact on the ball of their feet and then momentarily sag down on to their heel before an explosive toe-off.

VARIATIONS FROM NORMAL CONTACT PATTERNS

Joggers, just as walkers, with prolonged pronation problems which fail to allow for a normal resupination, will tend to contact on the whole pronated foot. Distance runners, who are fatigued towards the end of the race also may contact on their whole foot rather than going through a heel-foot-toe pattern. The whole foot contact has a disadvantage in that it does not allow for the normal eversion of the heel from a two-degree inverted position to a two-to-four degree pronated position (Figure 1). Thus, a great deal of meaningful shock absorption is lost.

Some distance runners attempt to run their entire race on the balls of their feet. This can lead to increased abnormal stress going through the foot and a jarring effect on the whole body.

The shorter distance runners must run on the balls of their feet to maintain the speed desirable for their events.

OTHER SPORTS

Almost all sports have some form of running involved. When one analyzes the sport, he notes that often times one foot is supinating as the other foot is pronating. Thus, in basketball, during the cutting maneuver the outside foot will be pronated while the inside foot is supinated. These same factors occur during skiing, football and in most all sports. Limitations of ranges of motion will affect the ability to carry out the individual movements necessary for each sport. High jumpers may have one problem with the take-off foot and another problem peculiar to the landing foot. Golfers may have a problem peculiar to their forward foot. Thus, it is essential to investigate the movements taking place in each sport and ascertain the various ranges of motion necessary for these sports. In any event, a biomechanically sound lower extremity will increase athletic efficiency and lessen the chance of injury in the sport.

SUMMARY

In summation, it can be seen that the biomechanically sound foot is the neutral foot. The neutral foot is that foot which would occur in a perfect foot during bipedal stance. This ideal foot is one in which the subtalar joint is neutral when the midtarsal joint is locked. During this situation all metatarsal heads rest firmly on the ground and the heel is perpendicular to the ground and parallel to long axis of the lower 1/3 of the leg. This neutral position should be present at the middle of mid-stance during walking or running. Failure to attain this neutral position with prolonged pronation prevents or retards normal resupination. Resupination is the key to a powerful toe-off with an efficient athletic stride. Inasmuch as it is generally estimated that at least 90% of our population has significant biomechanical variations from the ideal, it is understandable why so many athletes are becoming injured from overuse syndrome partially attributable to the unstable lower extremity. A stable lower extremity is biomechanically sound.

Chapter 5

Structural and Functional Lower Extremity Abnormalities Which Produce Abnormal Foot Function

INTRODUCTION

Abnormal function of the foot can occur from intrinsic as well as extrinsic problems. Intrinsic problems are those occurring within the foot and are by and large secondary to abnormal positioning of the joints within the foot. These are generally thought to be genetic traits. Extrinsic factors which effect foot function can be those of deviations in normal alignment of bones of the lower extremity as well as deviations from normal ranges of motions in the various joints of the lower extremity. Thus, there can be soft tissue influences which effect the normal function of the foot. These soft tissue limits of range of motion can be congenital or acquired. They may be acquired through some injury or neuromuscular disease as well as through improper training and conditioning. Improper training and conditioning can lead to dynamic muscle imbalances with tightness in some groups and more flexibility in other groups with alterations of motions.

It is generally preferable to speak in terms of the lower extremity in regards to the three cardinal body planes. We thus have deformities taking place on the transverse, frontal, and sagittal planes.

TRANSVERSE PLANE DEFORMITIES

Transverse plane deformities of the hip joint result in either increased internal or external rotation.[23] This can be a unilateral or bilateral problem. The main effect it has on the athlete is that varying contact angles of gait, which often times occur with compensating maneuvers, lower the efficiency of the athlete. Thus, an adducted (pigeon-toed) swing might cause the athlete to secondarily excessively pronate his foot at contact and precipitate the overuse syndromes which accompany abnormal pronation. The athlete with excessive external rotation of the hip joint would tend to contact on a pronated abducted foot. This type of foot tends to be nonpropulsive. Excessive adduction at contact may result in a criss-cross sway type gait which can lend itself to increased strain on the lateral hip stabilizers with hip pain and lateral thigh pain. This can also affect the knees.

The soft tissue range of motion limitations are easier to deal with than the osseous malpositions which occur within the hip joint or femur itself. The bones of the leg can be internally deviated due to a true torsion and respond poorly to physical attempts to increase the external malleolar position. Attempts to do so, in fact, may injure the knee joint.

The major problem with the adducted foot, secondary to an internal hip or leg deformity is that the athlete generally tries to straighten out the angle of gait by closed kinetic chain pronation. This uses up the pronation which is needed for normal contact. The foot itself may be adducted, secondary to metatarsus adductus. This type of foot is prone to a myriad of injuries. The athlete, often times, complains of pain over a prominent styloid process of the fifth metatarsal as well as pain over the lateral aspect of the fifth metatarsal head. The metatarsal phalangeal joints often times become unstable with attempts to accommodate to a conventional shoe. This may precipatate hallux valgus with bunion deformity and hammertoes.

FRONTAL PLANE DEFORMITIES

Frontal plane deformities include those of the femur, tibia, calcaneus, subtalar joint, and midtarsal joint.[23] At the hip joint, there can be either an increase or decrease in the declination angle of the head and neck of the femur as it meets the femoral shaft. This will result in either a knock-kneed or bow-legged deformity. Thus, there is a coxa-vara genu-valgum deformity with the knees together and tibial varum or a coxa-valgum genu-vara deformity with the knees apart and malleoli together (Figure 1). These frontal plane deformities tend to markedly alter the foot plant and side to side sway during running. In particular, we know that female athletes with a coxa-valga genu-vara tend to criss-cross on contact, instead of having a contact with the foot landing immediately upon the line of progression under the midline of the head. This allows for side-to-side sway with inefficiency and overuse syndrome.

The opposite of this deformity, which is the coxa-vara genu-valga, allows for contact on an everted heel and increases the pronatory strain of the foot. This results in severe strain on the medial aspect of the knee joint, as well as the ankle and subtalar joints.

FIGURE 1
FRONTAL PLANE DEFORMITIES OF THE LOWER EXTREMITIES

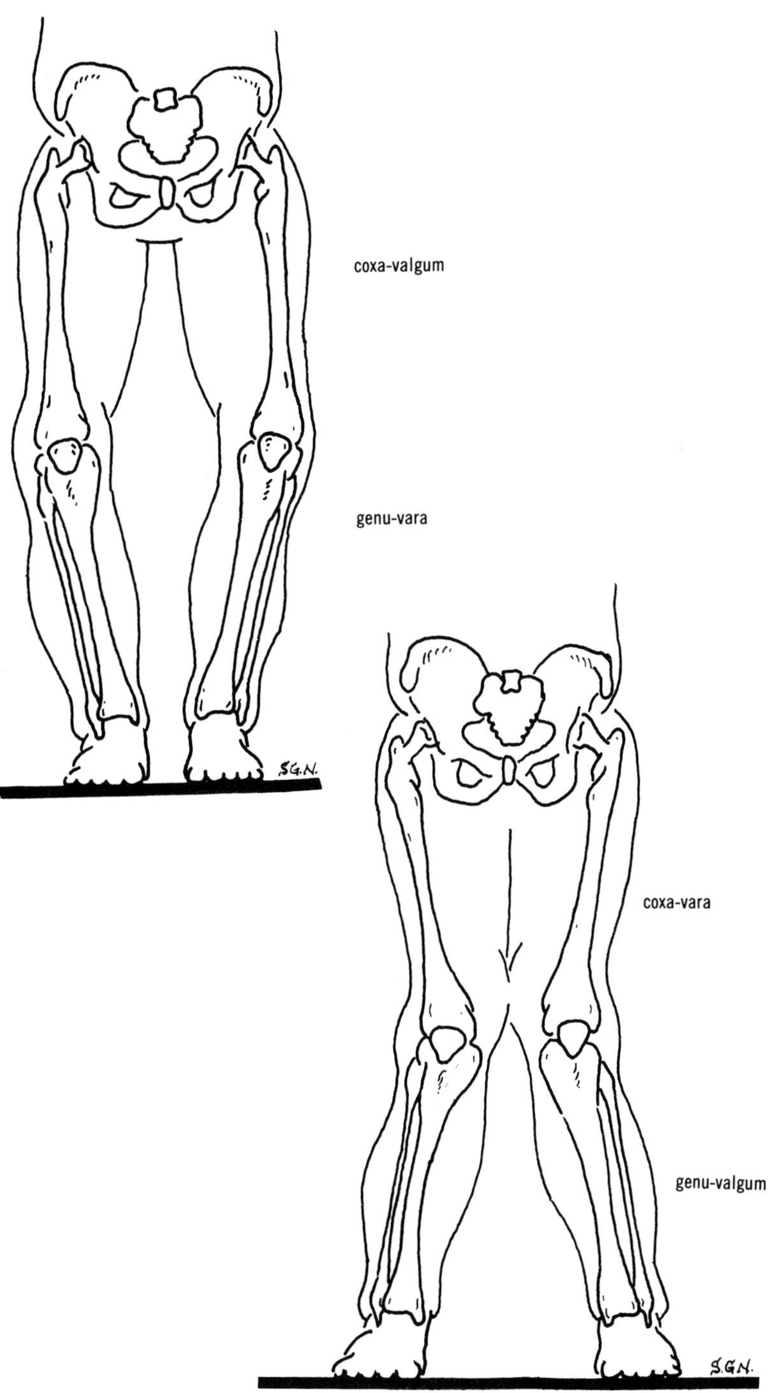

Tibial Varum

Bow legged deformity is usually referred to in medical terminology as tibial varum. In the case of tibial varum, the bisection of the lower 1/3 section of the tibia is in a varus attitude from the normal perpendicular attitude between the tibia and the supporting surface (Figure 2). In this case, the knees are far apart when the feet are together. This necessitates a pronation or eversion of the calcaneus to allow for normal foot function. Normal function usually occurs around a perpendicular heel bone position, but in the case of the tibial varum, at heel strike, there may be more than the four degrees of pronation taking place (Figure 3). This is necessary just to bring the calcaneus to a perpendicular position in relationship to the floor. This abnormal pronation results often times in symptoms in both the foot and the knee. The major symptoms taking place in the knee is termed "runner's knee"and is known as chondromalacia of the knee. More will be dealt with on this topic in another chapter.

FIGURE 2
TIBIAL VARUM

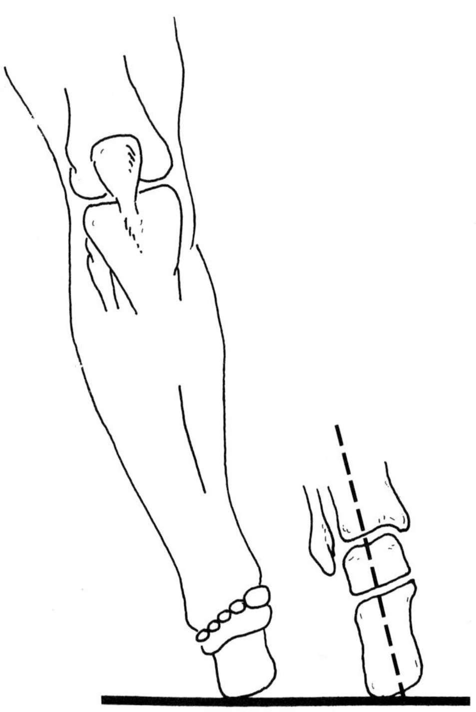

FIGURE 3
COMPENSATION FOR TIBIAL TORSION WITH LATERAL PATELLAR SUBLUXATIONS

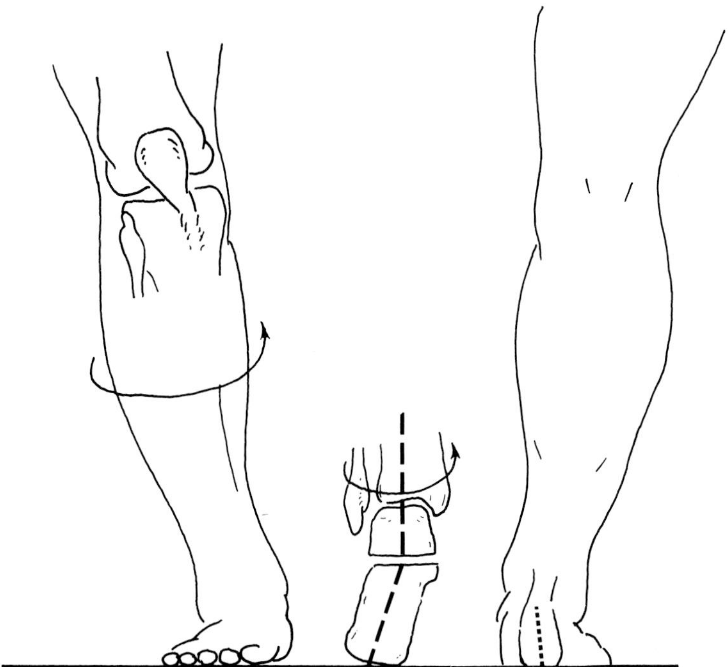

Associated with the tibial varum type deformity is the "pump bump".[40] Pump bumps or retro-calcaneal exostosis appear at the upper outer aspect of the heel bone and are attributed to abnormal pronation taking place at heel strike (Figure 4). Essentially, the calcaneus everts within the shoe causing the irritation. Initially, there is a blistering of the skin which is followed by fluid-filled sac or bursa forming underneath the skin. This bursa is usually painful and is complicated by the eventual overgrowth of the calcaneus beneath it. The tendo Achillis is often times inflamed along with this process as it rubs over the overgrowth of bone. The use of orthotics to control heel strike prevents this deformity from getting worse, although bony deposits, which have been laid down, usually do not go away. Along with the "pump bumps" and chondromalacia of the knee, shin splints can also occur, caused by abnormal heel strike pronation. All of these deformities are controlled by functional orthotics.[25, 29, 37]

FIGURE 4
RETROCALCANEAL EXOSTOSIS

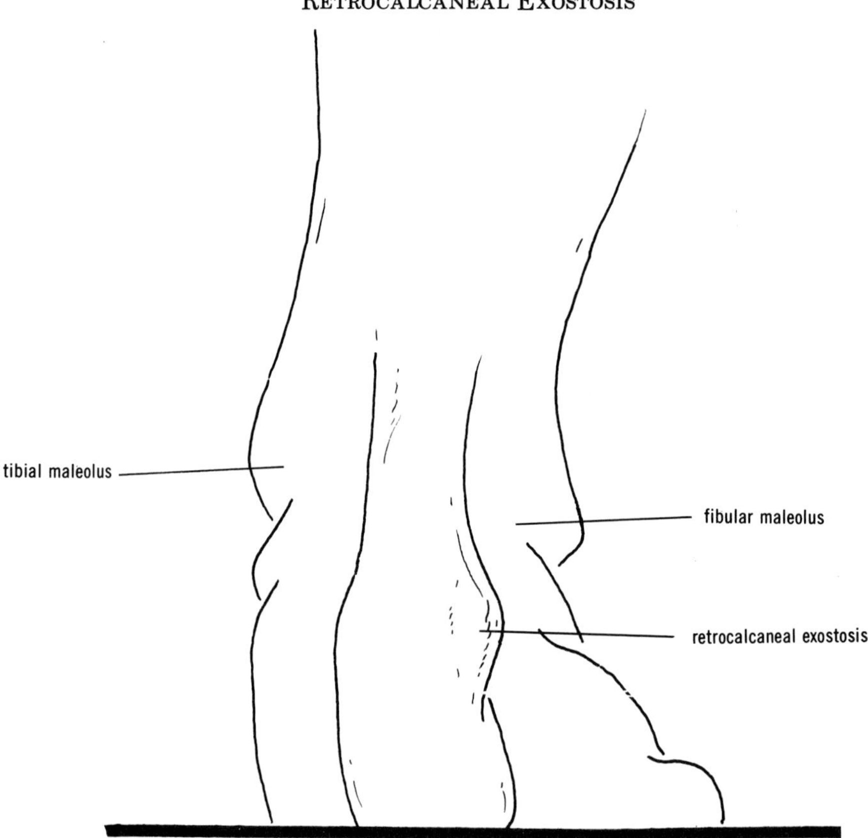

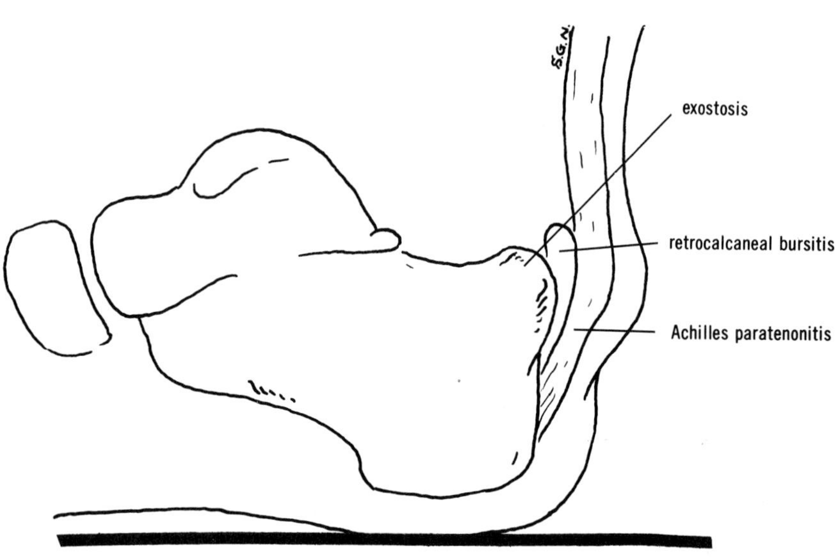

Subtalar Joint Varum

The subtalar joint, itself, may have a neutral position which is one which places the calcaneus in varus[22, 23] (Figure 5). The deformity termed here is subtalar joint varus. The varus neutral position of the subtalar joint creates problems similar to that of tibial varum. The calcaneus, itself, may have an osseus varus twist within it which allows for function similar to that seen with subtalar joint or tibial varum.

FIGURE 5
SUBTALAR VARUS AND COMPENSATION

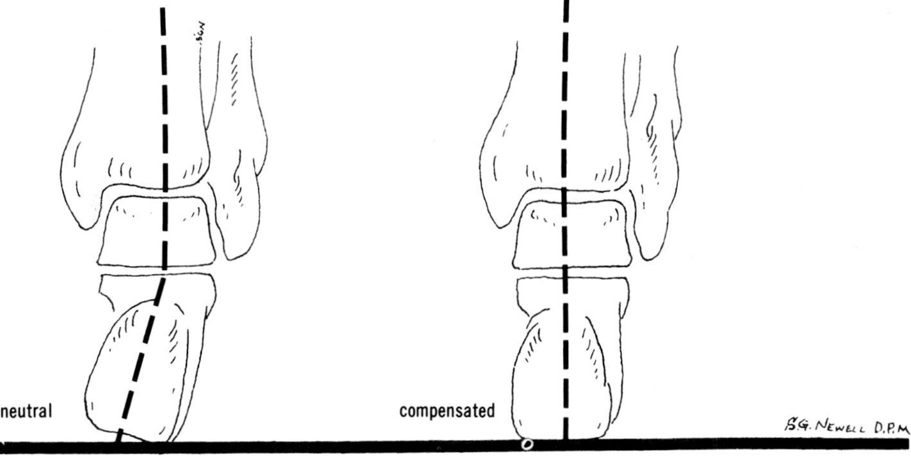

Midtarsal Joint Varus

The neutral position of the midtarsal joint can be structurally such that the locked midtarsal joint with the subtalar joint neutral, has the medial aspect of the foot raised and not in contact with the weight-bearing surface. This is termed "forefoot varus" (Figure 6). The opposite of this deformity is the maximally pronated midtarsal joint having a valgus relationship with the calcaneus[22, 23, 29] (Figure 7). Both these deformities lend themselves to various postural symptoms and eventual osseus malpositions. Forefoot varus and valgus will be dealt with in more detail in later chapters.

FIGURE 6
FOREFOOT VARUS AND COMPENSATION

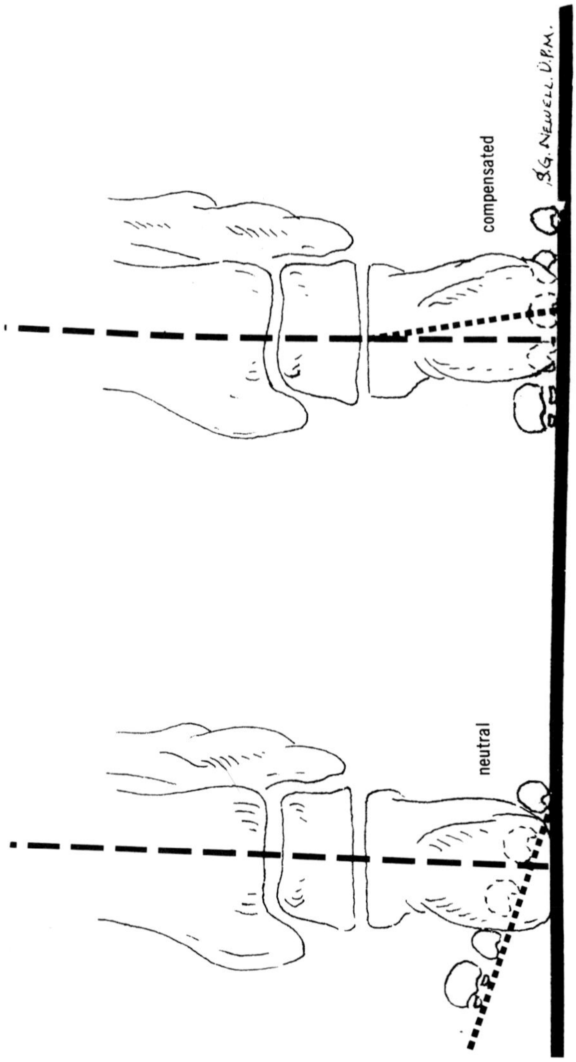

FIGURE 7
FOREFOOT VALGUS AND COMPENSATION

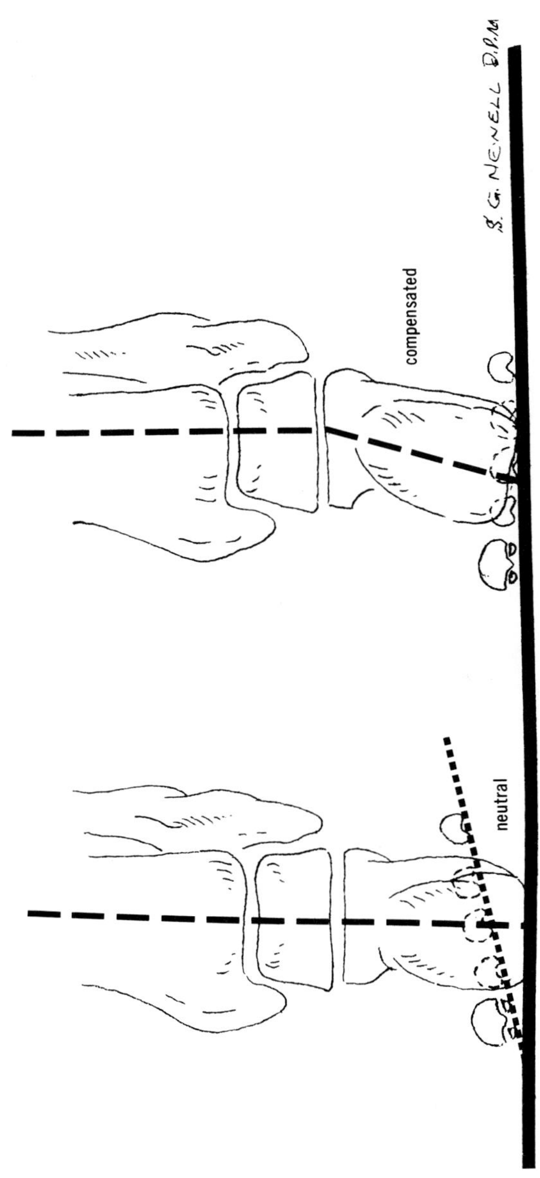

SAGITTAL PLANE DEFORMITIES

The major sagittal plane deformities which affect athletes are those of an unstable knee joint with hyperextension as well as an ankle joint and or forefoot equinus condition. In addition, there are various forms of excessive pronated feet or high arched cavus feet which could be classified as sagittal plane deformities. Hyperextension of the knee may be secondary to an equinus deformity of the lower extremity and makes the knee more prone to injury. This will be dealt with in greater detail in other sections.

The Ankle Joint

At the middle of the stance phase of gait, the tibia moves forward about ten degrees over the talar dome of the foot. There must be enough motion present at the ankle joint to allow for this forward migration of the tibia. If this motion is prevented by either a tight gastrocnemius or soleus muscle, or osseous limitations within the joint itself, then a compensatory unlocking of the subtalar joint with secondary collapse of the forefoot must occur (Figure 8). With unlocking of the subtalar joint the midtarsal joint becomes mobile and dorsi and plantarflexion can take place around the oblique midtarsal joint axis. This ten degrees of dorsiflexion of the foot upon the leg must occur and if it is not occurring at the ankle joint, it will occur within the foot or at the knee. When lack of motion at the ankle is absorbed at the knee it is manifested by an athlete performing with a flexed knee position.[32, 33]

FIGURE 8
EQUINUS DEFORMITY

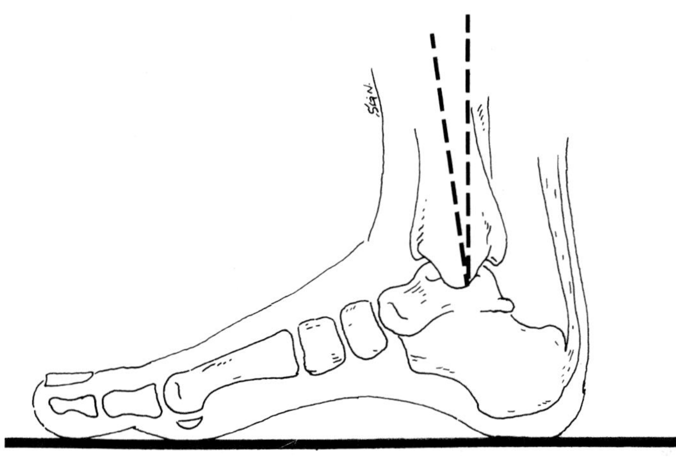

NEUTRAL FOOT

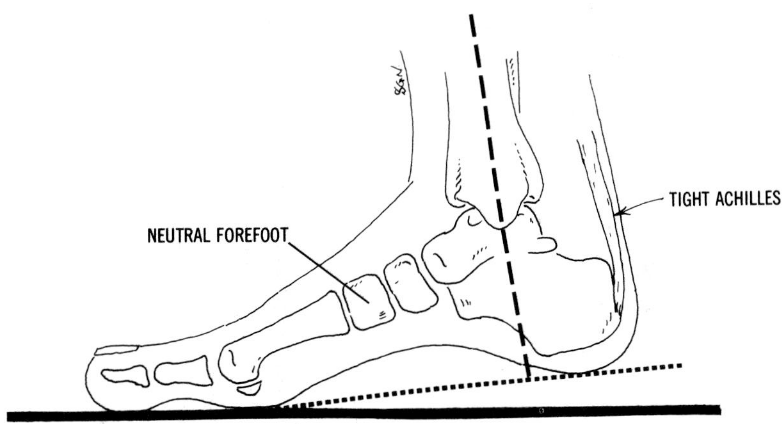

NORMAL DORSIFLEXION

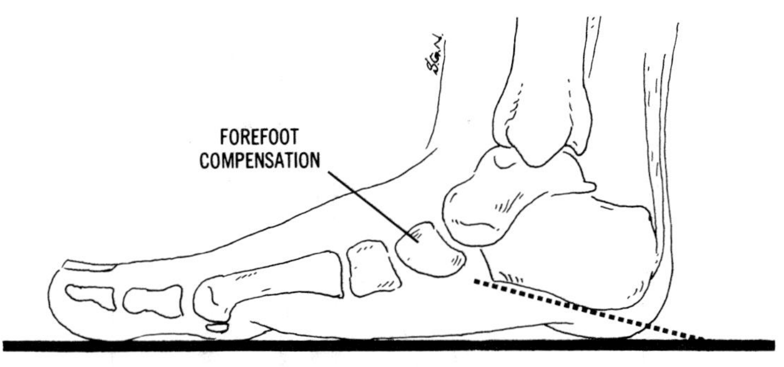

ABNORMAL DORSIFLEXION

FIGURE 9
FLEXIBLE ANTERIOR EQUINUS

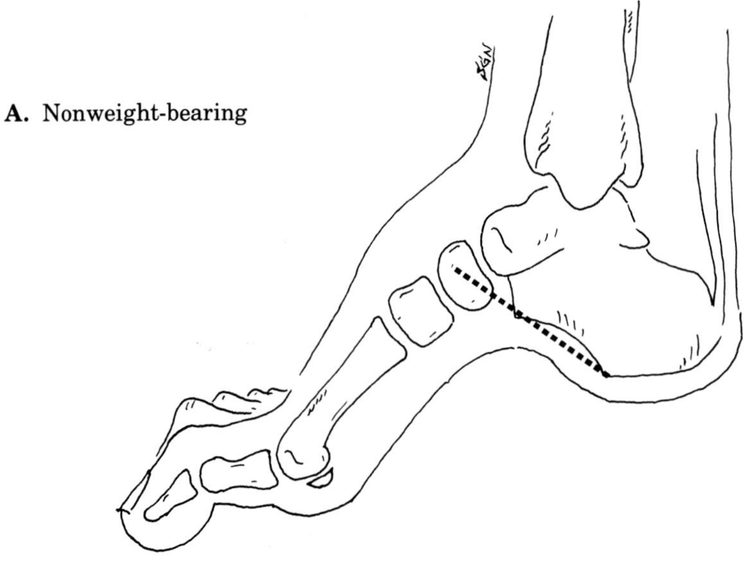

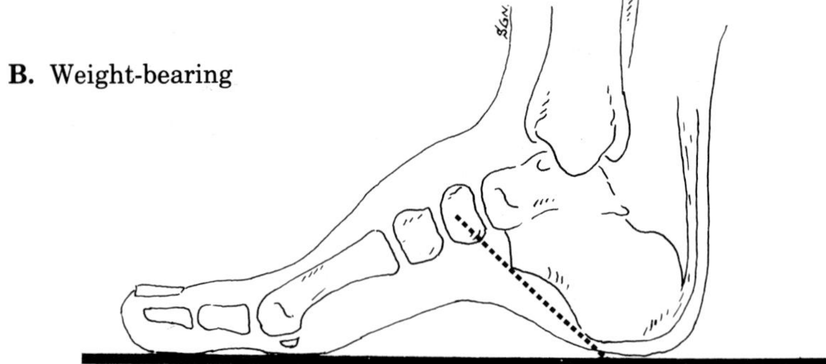

The compensatory pronation of the foot secondary to the equinus condition, that condition which is a lack of the normal ten degrees of dorsiflexion of the neutral foot upon the leg, results in extensive symtoms, such as medial arch pain, plantar fasciitis, posterior leg fatigue, as well as a multiple of bony abnormalities of the foot, including bunions, hammertoes, and tailor's bunions. In addition, overuse symptoms are grossly exaggerated with the gastrocnemius or soleus equinus deformity.[32]

Functional (Runner's) Equinus

It is not uncommon for the gastrocnemius muscles to be tight in an athlete if he is not training or conditioning himself properly. Runners tend to overdevelop their posterior muscles to the detriment of the anterior antagonistic muscles. Thus, upon initial examination the runner may have what appears to be mild tightness of the gastrocsoleus group with the knee extended. This will be found to disappear with proper stretching exercises. A soleus equinus may be present when there is limitation of dorsiflexion with both the extended and flexed knee position.

Anterior Equinus (Forefoot Equinus)

The anterior equinus type foot is one with a very high arch[26] (Figure 9). Usually in this foot the plane of the forefoot is plantar to the plane of the rearfoot and this is evident in the nonweight bearing attitude. This is the cavus type foot with a very high calcaneal inclination angle which has its main problem in the lack of shock absorption. The range of motion of the subtalar joint is usually limited and there is very poor contact shock absorption properties. These patients have a great deal of problems with pain under the metatarsal heads as well as plantar fascial strains.[38]

SUMMARY

In conclusion, we have presented the various structural and functional abnormalities which effect normal foot function. It is important to be able to examine the athlete and determine the degrees of deformities taking place at the various levels of the lower extremity. The significance of the various biomechanical abnormalities will be discussed in further chapters.

Chapter 6

Overuse Syndrome of the Foot and Leg

INTRODUCTION

Thus far in this book, we have stressed the normal functioning of the foot as well as abnormal function and structure which produce symptoms in the athlete. This chapter will concentrate on the overuse syndrome and those symptoms which accompany this condition. Malfunction of the lower extremity can well occur from biomechanical abnormalities of the lower extremity as well as biomechanical malfunctioning of the lower extremity secondary to dynamic muscle imbalance as well as overuse. Normal function depends upon (1) normal lower extremity biomechancial function and structure, (2) proper conditioning, (3) proper training. Proper biomechanical function and structure depend on balanced muscle strength as well as control of structural abnormalities of the lower extremity utilizing functional foot orthotics. Proper conditioning depends upon balanced muscle strength. Proper training depends upon adapting to stressful situations without plunging into an overstress situation. Strength, as well as flexibility, is paramount for the proper function. This chapter will concentrate on those overuse syndromes which accompany structural abnormalities as well as improper conditioning and training. [29, 37]

SYMPTOMS OF THE OVERUSE SYNDROME

Training is basically preparing the body to adapt to stressful situations. Athletic competition is stressful. When there is more stress that the body is accustomed to tolerating, the symptoms of overuse begin. These symptoms initially present themselves as nagging, bothersome aches and pains. There may be a dull ache in the arch of one foot and in the knee of the other foot. When these symptoms first occur, they generally cause difficulty only after competition or a brisk workout. The symptoms become more intense about an hour after athletic endeavors. Initially, these injuries are only bothersome and the athlete continues to train and compete. As the athlete continues to place his body under conditions of undue stress, these injuries can progress from the *first stage* of being only bothersome, to the *second stage* of being moderately severe.

The *second stage* overuse symptoms are essentially those of pain during, as well as after, athletic activities. These pains gradually increase from day to day and the athlete becomes worried about them. There may be a tendo Achillis problem which limits the athlete to running only on flat surfaces. There may be a knee problem which limits the basketball player from rebounding. There may be a posterior tibial tendon or muscle inflammation which prevents the tennis player from rushing the net. Grade 2 injuries become severe without proper treatment and rest and will often progress to *grade 3 overuse* symptoms.

Grade three symptoms are associated with pain before, during, and after even modest activities. Normal athletic participation is impossible. Pain is present even with walking and possibly during rest. The athlete is totally unable to train and the injury will respond only to rest and medical care.

The significance of these three stages of overuse syndrome is that the grade one injuries respond rapidly to a biomechanical and functional approach and the athlete can continue with training and competition after a relatively short period of rehabilitation. The grade two injuries take more time to recuperate from and permanent chronic damage may be precipitated. The grade three injuries take a great deal of rest and rehabilitation and more serious injury, with chronic fibrosis or arthritis, may be anticipated.[29] Once a grade two or three injury is present, there is always that chance for recurrence despite the most rational biomechanical and functional approach to the problem.

The first general warning signs to the athlete that may accompany these overuse symptoms are those of generalized lethargy, which may be accompanied by a mild sore throat or cold. The athlete will feel stiffness all over, with generalized aches and pains. There may be lack of a desire to train. There will be concern on the part of the athlete that a seemingly mild injury is getting worse rather than better. When any of these symptoms are present, the overuse problem is evident and treatment is necessary to prevent further injury. Treatment consists of proper biomechanical function, training, and conditioning. Proper training must include sensible rest periods.

OVERUSE SYNDROMES SECONDARY TO BIO-MECHANICAL ABNORMALITIES OF THE LOWER EXTREMITY

Those biomechanical structural abnormalities of the lower extremity which can produce injury and overuse syndrome have already been discussed. In review, we know that there may be tibial valgum or tibial varum which contributes to overuse syndromes of the foot and leg. Subtalar joint varum and valgum may also contribute to lower extremity problems. The midtarsal joint may have a neutral position which is fixed in varum or valgum and which precludes to a myriad of foot, leg, and knee problems. We have discussed the importance of the high arch and the low arch foot in regard to foot problems. Further correlations between feet types and overuse syndrome will be discussed in Chapter Seven.

Deviations from normal structure place abnormal stresses upon the body. Electromyographic studies show that increased intrinsic musculature activity with prolonged, abnormal pronation, is present.[38] Excessive pronation can lead to shin splints of the posterior group with prolonged phasic activity. Abnormal contact can lead to anterior muscle group problems as they function out of phase to decelerate an overstriding foot.

CONDITIONING AND ITS RELATIONSHIP TO THE OVERUSE SYNDROME

Conditioning problems are secondary to overspecialization of muscles. Long-distance runners overspecialize in their posterior muscle groups. They have tight tendo Achillis, as well as hamstring muscles. There is a dynamic imbalance between the anterior and posterior muscle groups. The anterior leg muscle groups are characteristically weak as are the quadricep muscles. This is one of the reasons that long-distance runners get anterior muscle group shin splints as well as knee problems secondary to improper patellar function with weak quadicep muscles. The treatment for these imbalance problems is to develop both strength and flexibility. Isometric and isotonic contractions are necessary for developing the strength of the weakened muscle groups and at the same time flexibility and gradual stretching exercises must be utilized to keep all muscles lengthened and supple. Flexibility exercises are necessary before, and even more important after, workouts and training.[7] Running makes muscles tight and it is very necessary to stretch these tightened structures after running activities.

We notice that sprinters have very strong quadricep muscles as well as tight hamstrings and posterior leg muscles. Their injuries are more overstrain than overstress injuries as they explode from the starting blocks during races. Their need for flexibility, as well as strength, cannot be overstressed.

Proper conditioning should include bent-knee sit-ups, to develop the anterior muscle groups of the abdomen, which help

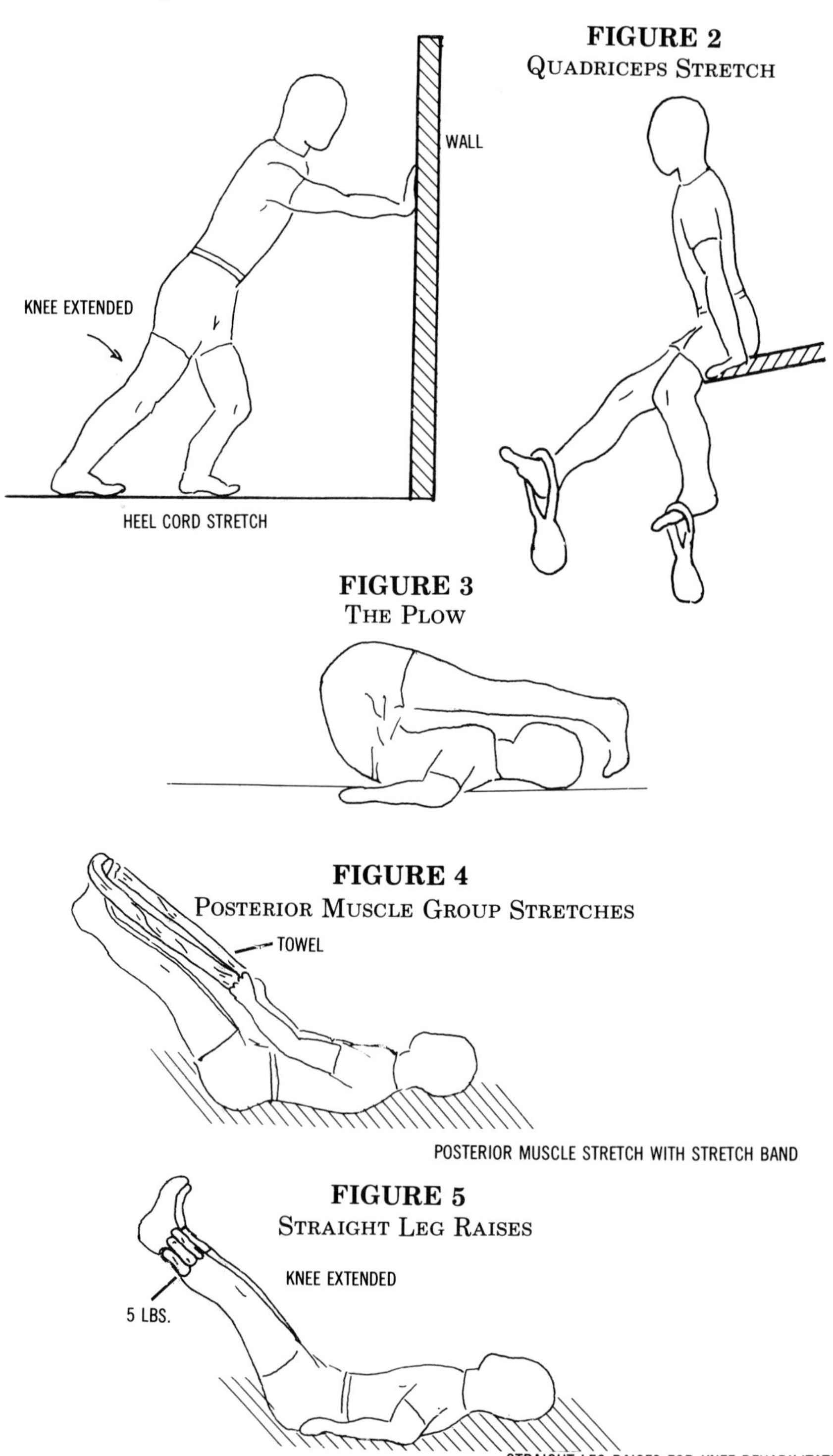

FIGURE 1
Static Stretch of Posterior Muscle Group

FIGURE 2
Quadriceps Stretch

FIGURE 3
The Plow

FIGURE 4
Posterior Muscle Group Stretches

FIGURE 5
Straight Leg Raises

keep the back in alignment and allow for a normal upright running stride. Conditioning of the thighs should include quadricep stretches, as well as isometric contraction sets. Straight-leg raises are always good for the thighs. The hips are kept in condition by front, side and back leg raises carried out at least twenty times a day. The knees are kept in good condition by isometric, quadricep contractions with a set of twenty contractions held for twenty seconds, twice daily. In addition, straight leg raises with gradual increases of weight on the foot to five pounds are very useful. The various joints are maintained with range of motion, flexibility, and strength exercises. These include heel, toe, medial foot, and lateral foot raises. Nonweight-bearing foot exercises include making circles starting from a small circumference to a large circumference. The ankles are conditioned by gentle yoga type stretching with each stretch being held a minimum of thirty seconds. This invokes the reverse myotatic response.[7] Sudden bouncy type stretching activity is not beneficial and may strain muscles and tendons.

Ankles are rehabilitated for kinesthetic sensation, following sprains, by bouncing a ball against the wall while hopping on one leg. This has been shown to greatly reduce the talar tilt following severe ankle sprains. The feet are kept in condition by doing toe curls, as well as arch lifts (Figures 1-5).

PROPER TRAINING TO PREVENT THE OVERUSE SYNDROME

The overuse syndrome often times occurs when the runner has the attitude that if five miles a day makes me a good runner, then ten miles a day will make me a great runner. Although this concept may be true, the runner cannot jump from five miles a day to ten miles a day without a gradual period of buildup. The body must gradually be conditioned to accept more stress. This stress includes being able to handle glycogen depletion in the muscles, as well as increased aerobic states during explosive activities. The body must slowly adapt to increases in stress. Although a runner may do quite well on only three miles a day even with minimum to moderate biomechanical abnormalities, a jump to six miles a day may very well bring about overuse syndromes and injuries which will need functional orthotics as well as proper conditioning and training to reverse.

Other examples of improper training include sudden changes in terrain. A beginning athlete may do most of his training on a flat surface and then begin running on hills to develop strength. This may place muscles under an abnormal stretch and often times creates tendo Achillis problems. Sudden changes in running speed may cause rupture of muscle groups. Changes from training shoes with a shock absorbing sole to racing flats with hardly any sole at all may cause considerable problems. This problem may be secondary to lack of absorbing properties in the shoe as well as to the lower heel which places the posterior muscle groups under increased stress. Basic rules of training and racing are often times violated. An athlete may usually participate for three times the average daily training time and distance. There should be at least 40 hours rest after a hard workout. There should be from one week to one month of rest from rigorous competition after a very hard race, as in the case of a marathon. Shorter races require shorter periods of rest.[29]

Proper training, then, requires varied workouts alternating between hard and easy sessions. Proper training should include gradual changes of terrain from hard surfaces to soft surfaces. There should be proper conditioning integrated with training with emphasis on flexibility and strength exercises for at least ten minutes before and after every workout session. Proper training must include gradual increases in the amount of stress if the body is expected to adapt without injury.

An example is in the beginning jogger. The beginning jogger should walk briskly for about two hundred hards followed by an interval of jogging for another two hundred yards. This workout should be gradually increased until the jogger can go for a mile without being out of breath or overly tired. The jogging should be for no more than five out of the seven weekly days. On the rest days, the jogger may ride a bike for gentle relaxation and exercise. The jogger might increase his distance from one mile to two miles over a period of one month by gradually adding increases in the distance.

An example of this would be going one mile one day, a mile and a half on the next day, back to one mile and one and one half the next. On the following week, the runner might go one mile, one and one half, one mile and then two miles, until his distance is gradually increased.

OVERUSE SYNDROMES

We have discussed the overuse syndrome of the lower extremity in regard to their etiologies. We will now consider the various parts of the lower extremity and discuss those symptoms which are often found.

Back

The back may be affected by low back strain, as well as sciatica. These problems often occur secondary to asymmetry to the lower extremity.[34] This will be discussed in Appendix 2. These problems may also occur secondary to overuse symptoms and in particular, chronic pronation of the feet.[25, 34] The low back pain may be a nagging type ache at the L-5, S-1 or L-4, L-5 area or may be painful around the sacroiliac joints secondary to overuse. These may be sharp pains radiating behind the gluteals then medially in the thigh and leg secondary to sciatic nerve involvement. When sciatica is present there will be increased pain with straight leg raises.

Conservative treatment for sciatica and low back pain consists of a biomechanical approach to any lower extremity abnormality, as well as bent knee sit-ups to help strengthen the anterior aspect of the low back. Functional, anatomical, or combination asymmetrics of the pelvis as well as increased lordosis secondary to abnormal pronation must be corrected.

Hip

Overuse syndromes of the hip include tensor fascial latae strains, as well as hip pointers. These injuries often occur when running on slanting roads which place these structures under unusual strain. The hip pointers are painful areas at the anterior, superior iliac crest.[21] The tensor fascial lateral strains are palpable painful rifts of the lateral thigh. The iliotibial band may "snap" over the greater trochanter of the femur with a secondary adventitious bursitis. This is often associated with abnormal lower extremity structure, as well as improper training an muscle imbalance.

Treatment consists of correcting biomechanic and soft tissue imbalances. An adventitious bursitis will respond well to physical therapy, as well as a local cortico-steroid injection.

Buttocks

Centered around the buttocks are complaints associated with adventitious bursitis, as well as ischial tuberosity tendonitis and periostitis. These are problems secondary to overstrain, as when the athlete changes from the flats to the hills. They can be sometimes related to abnormal biomechanical structure and functions. Treatment consists of physical therapy and functional control.

Thigh

Medial hamstrings pulls are common in the thigh in sprinters as well as long-distance runners. These usually respond well to icing for the first 48 hours, as well as gentle stretching exercises during the rehabilitative period.

Knee

Chondromalacia and related patellar malfunction syndromes are the primary noncollision knee injuries. These malfunctions are related to improper functioning of the foot, as well as weak quadricep muscles, and intrinsic knee joint instability.[2, 16, 21, 24, 35, 29] Knee problems will be discussed in further detail in Chapter 14.

In addition to patellar malfunction problems, are those of bursitis and tendonitis of the medial and lateral hamstrings as they insert around the knee joint. There may also be medial meniscal problems which sometimes respond to a biomechanical approach. These problems should be distinguished from patellar symptoms, inasmuch as they may be in need of a referral to an orthopedic specialist if they fail to respond to conservative treatment.

Treatment of overuse knee problems should, at first, be conservative and centered around a proper restoration of muscle functioning including the quadriceps and medial and lateral hamstrings. Functional foot control must be obtained. It is imperative to have proper foot functioning before conservative treatment for any knee problem can be adequately evaluated.

Returning to activity following patellar malfunction may be quite frustrating. A basic rule that I use is that if there is no pain before or during activity, but some pain after activity and functional control has been accomplished, activity may be continued. As soon as there is any knee pain related to activity, then the athlete must ease back and rest. Alternative sports may be utilized while rehabilitating the patient. Swimming and bike riding are good alternatives. Those activities which require stressful flexion of the knee should be avoided. The importance of quadricep exercises and orthotics for total rehabilitation cannot be overstressed.

Leg

Overuse syndromes of the leg include soft tissue as well as bony problems. I have had many cases of stress fractures of the leg. Stress fractures of the tibia, in runners, seem to occur more often in the proximal quarter. Those of the fibula occur more often in the lower quarter. Soft tissue injuries of the leg are further discussed Chapter 15. These include the myositis, periostitis and tendonitis problems of all four muscular compartments of the leg. When the flexor group is involved, there is often a posterior tibial or flexor digitorum longus shin splint type syndrome secondary to overstress and overuse during midstance and propulsion. When the anterior muscle group is involved, there are shin splint symptoms which occur during heel contact. Both of these problems are secondary to a combination of overuse, overstress and improper foot functioning. Treatment consists of evaluating and treating the actual etiologies.

The same basic principles apply to these injuries as to all injuries — that of restoring proper foot function, as well as adhering to proper conditioning and training.[21]

Ankle Joint and Subtalar Joint

The ankle and subtalar joints may be involved secondary to what I have termed "the chronic pronatory syndrome." This consists of a compression of the lateral aspect of the rearfoot, with a tension over the medial aspect of the rearfoot. This leads to a peroneal tendonitis on the lateral aspect of the foot, as well as sural nerve compression and entrapment. Tension occurs over the tarsal tunnel area and may result in a tarsal tunnel syndrome. There may also be traction upon the medial calcaneal nerve with increased pronation. The medial plantar nerve can furthermore become entrapped in an adventitious bursa of the heel. It is often referred to as a stone bruise. The chronic pronation syndrome may also include posterior tibial tendonitis at the medial aspect of the ankle which may migrate proximally and become a chronic posterior muscle group myositis or shin splint. (See Chapter 15.)

The chronic pronation syndrome responds well to a biomechanical approach with functional orthotics. Injections may be necessary, using local anesthetic and cortico-steroids when the sinus tarsi is painful or where adventitious bursitis or long-standing tendonitis is present. This may only be done for chronic problems when the functional approach is also being taken.

Heel

The heel presents itself with overuse syndromes of the retrocalcaneal area, as well as the heel spur area. The retrocalcaneal bursitis exostosis and secondary tendo Achillis tendonitis is well known. This occurs secondary to excessive abnormal contacts stress as well as midstance overstress.

Calcaneal problems may be accentuated by hill running. Heel spur problems fall into the *chronic pronatory syndrome* category and are treated by functional control, as well as appropriate injections. Heel spurs which are long-standing and fail to respond to any other form of treatment may have to be surgically excised, at which time the plantar fascia is also released.

Retrocalcaneal exostoses are treated with orthotics in the early stages to reduce contact pronation. Chronic exostoses may require surgical excision.

Plantar Aspect of the Foot

The plantar aspect of the foot is plagued with overuse syndromes including fasciitis, myositis, and abductor strains. These problems are secondary to prolonged abnormal pronation and respond to correction of this problem. In addition, the medial aspect of the arch may have a chronic strain, which also responds to functional control.

Forefoot

Overuse syndromes of the forefoot include the plantar interdigital neuromas. These appear to be caused by improper metatarsal head functioning, which may be secondary to abnormal pronation. Neuromas are also aggravated by the overstress which accompanies prolonged training. Following excessive athletic endeavors, there is an increase in plantar metatarsal head capsulitis, as well as bursitis. The forefoot may be also plagued with extensor tendonitis and various blisters, corns, and calluses. Under metatarsal heads there are calluses which may progress to intractable plantar keratomas with bursitis. On the medial plantar aspect of the foot, tibial sesamoidities is not uncommon following long athletic endeavors. Tailor's bunions are often times aggravated by tight fitting shoes, ski boots, or prolonged athletic endeavors. This also holds true for hammertoes and bunions. Bunions and digital deformities may be a direct sequella of prolonged chronic pronation.

SUMMARY

The importance of the overuse syndrome has been stressed. Unaccustomed overstress leads to overuse which leads to injury. Injury may be secondary to (1) improper biomechanical structure or function, (2) improper training, (3) improper conditioning. All three factors must be considered when treating athletic injury. The most common athletic injuries are those of overuse. The warning signs of overuse were stressed and they must be well heeded by all athletes. It is encouraging that the biomechanical approach to injury appears to work well. It is also necessary to realize that preventive biomechanical treatment is often times the athlete's best insurance to not getting injured.

Chapter 7

Foot Types and Injury Predilections

INTRODUCTION

Basic foot types exist and generalizations as to predisposition for certain overuse injuries associated with a particular foot type are useful. I prefer to classify feet as to calcaneal neutral position, calcaneal everted position, and calcaneal inverted position. The distinguishing features of these three classifications appear to be in the subtalar joint neutral position, stance position, and total range of motion. The associated foot types are respectively neutral, pronated, and cavus. Midtarsal joint neutral position and rigidity, as well as the amount of tibial varum or valgum, effect the calcaneal stance position and contribute to the end resultant foot type.

THE AVERAGE SPORTS MEDICINE PATIENT

The average sports medicine patient seen in my office, over the past four years, has been between the ages of twelve and fifty. The oldest is seventy-three and still an active runner. Over one thousand long-distance runners have been treated and a number of participants in tennis, field-hockey, basketball, softball, gymnastics, race-walking, and football. We have seen several skiers whose foot problems are often related to their wide feet being forced into narrow, rigid ski boots. Some of the skiers also have leg and foot problems secondary to biomechanical problems (See Appendix 1). Most of these athletes had very few problems associated with their everyday activities; most of their symptoms were secondary to malfunction during athletic participation. Those with the more severe foot deformities did, however, as expected, have problems with and without athletic endeavors.

SURVEY OF BIOMECHANICAL MEASUREMENTS

A survey of these patients revealed that the average subtalar joint total range of motion was 28 degrees (Figure 1). The neutral subtalar joint position was in two to three degrees of varus. This allowed for 21 degrees of supination and seven degrees of pronation. Most of these patients have from two to four degrees of tibial varum. The midtarsal joint range of motion averaged five to six degrees of varus. The ankle joint initially had between eight and twelve degrees of dorsiflexion. Almost all of the athletes had *at least* ten degrees of dorsiflexion following good stretching exercises. All of the athletes had tight hamstrings and most of the long-distance runners had weak quadriceps. The average angle of gait was between four to ten degrees abducted. It is apparent that the average foot seen in patients that had no symptoms during normal activity, but only symptoms during jogging and running activities is indeed somewhat different from the ideal normal as explained in Chapter 4. The *ideal* normal foot would have a range of motion of about thirty degrees total, with no subtalar joint varus or valgus.

Some trends were noted in regard to foot types and success at various events. It was noted that the better long-distance runners often times had narrower ranges of motion and more rigid feet than the average long-distance runner. This was just a trend, inasmuch as some outstanding long-distance runners and marathoners had extremely pronated feet which appeared to be very ill-suited for their type of sport.

VARIATIONS FROM THE AVERAGE FOOT TYPE

As the neutral stance position of the calcaneus varies from the ideal perpendicular to the average three to four degree everted calcanaal stance position, more symptoms appeared to be prevalent in the athlete. These symptoms increase in severity and in frequency as the calcaneal bipedal stance position becomes more and more everted. Those symptoms were those of the flexible pronated foot. On the other hand, the calcaneal stance position may become inverted and range from a perpendicular position to one of varus. In these instances, different types of overuse symptoms are more prevalent than with the flexible pronated foot.

FIGURE 1

Foot Types with Subtalar Joint Ranges of Motion

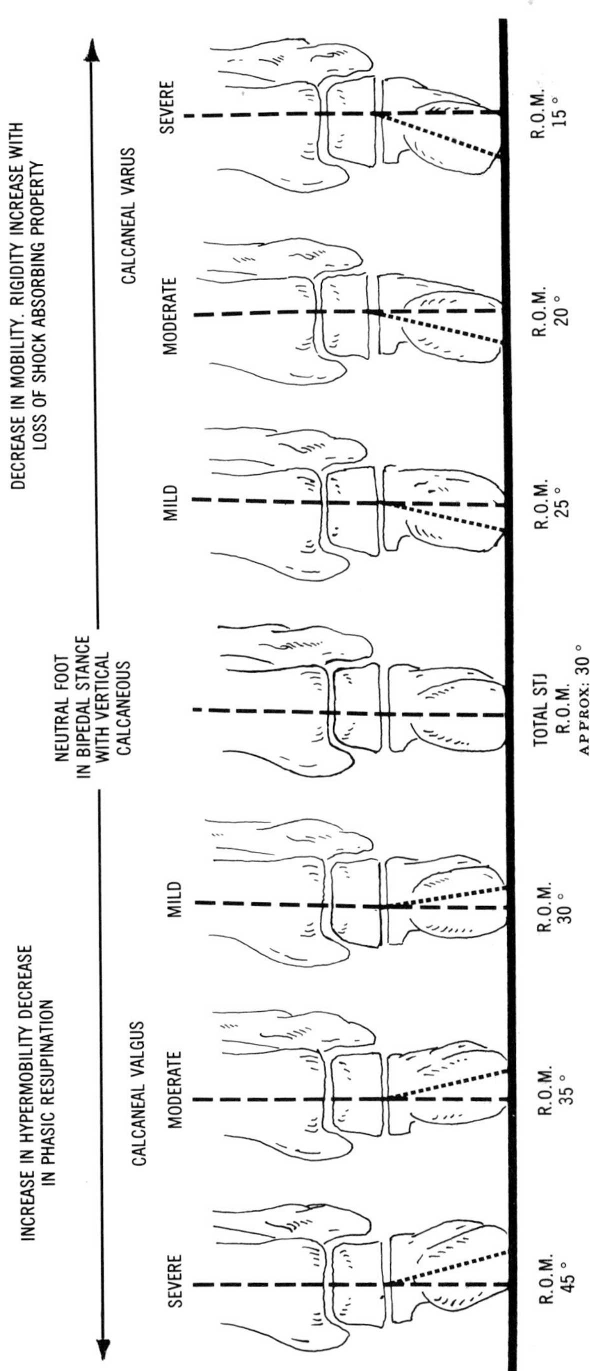

As a trend, the more rigid feet seen had a higher arch, a more narrow subtalar joint range of motion with a varus neutral position, and very limited calcaneal eversion past the perpendicular. The more flexible flat feet have a greater subtalar joint range of motion with a forefoot varus and increased calcaneal valgus. As the calcaneal stance position becomes more everted, the severity and the likelihood of pronatory overuse syndromes increases. As the calcaneal stance position becomes more perpendicular and then finally varus, those symptoms secondary to poor shock absorbing properties of the foot with increased contact stress tend to become more prevalent and severe. Stress fractures may occur (Figure 1).

Of course, flexible flat feet may become statically deformed secondary to subluxations and arthritic changes.[33] These rigid flat feet, while functioning maximally pronated, lack good shock absorbing properties. This is also true of the fully compensated pronated type foot which occurs quite often with equinus deformity. This foot type may still be flexible in its earlier stages, yet has no contact pronation, inasmuch as the calcaneus never resupinates. It has been observed that flexible foot deformities, when treated early in life, respond well without the deformity progressing to the more rigid stages. The cavus type foot, however, even with early instituted treatment, may progress to more rigid states. Conservative treatment does appear to slow down this progression while it usually helps the symptoms presenting with the cavus deformity. I will discuss first those feet which are pronated and then those feet which appear to be more rigid with a higher arch.

The Mildly Pronated Foot

The mildly pronated foot has a calcaneal stance position of about four to six degrees of valgus (Figures 1 and 2). This foot presents with a mild forefoot deformity of about four to six degrees. There may be two to four degrees of tibial varum present. The amount of tibial varum will, of course, effect the calcaneal stance position, inasmuch as subtalar joint pronation will be necessary to compensate for tibial varum. When combined, rearfoot varus and forefoot varus deformities are present, combinations of overuse symptoms appear (Figure 3).

ANTERIOR POSTERIOR XRAY OF NEUTRAL FOOT WITH CONGRUENT MIDTARSAL JOINT

FIGURE 2A

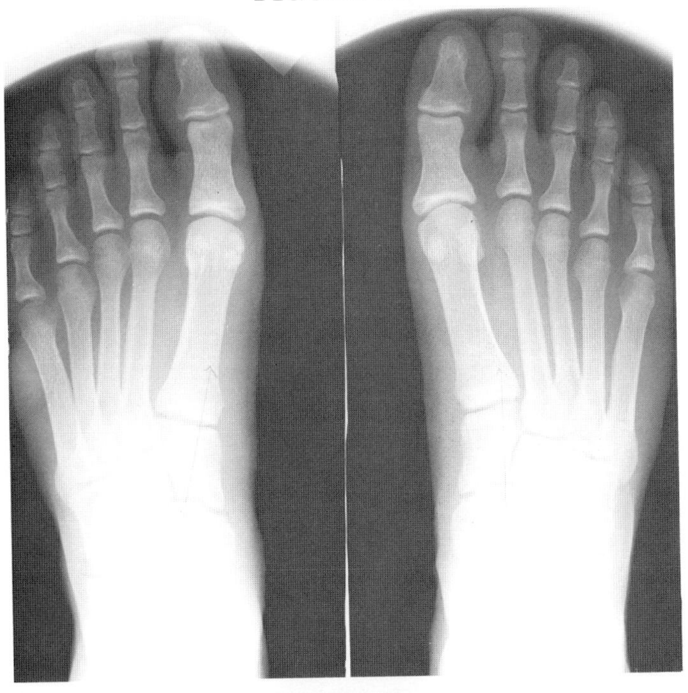

FIGURE 2B

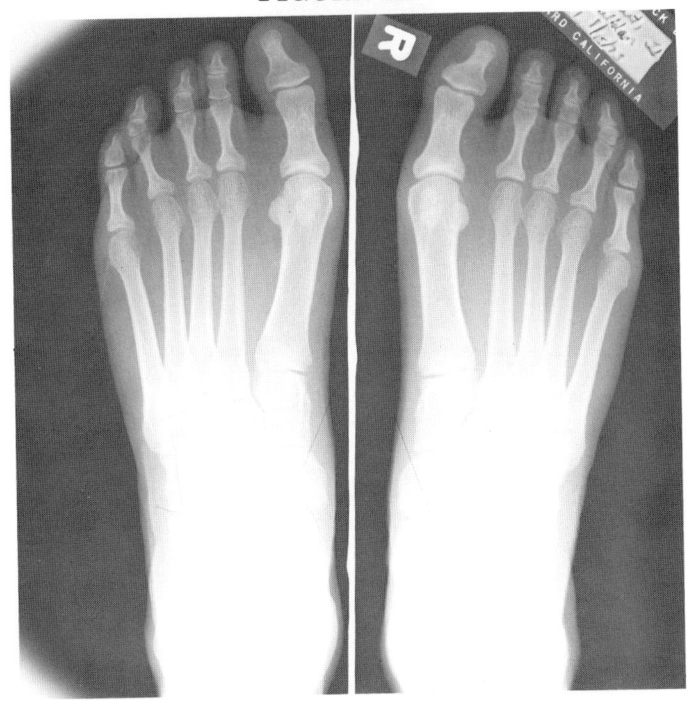

Those symptoms associated with the forefoot varus type deformity are those of posterior tibial muscle myositis and tendonitis, as well as generalized shin splints. Along with this, there is a tendency towards chondromalacia and related disorders of the knee. Younger children may present Osgood-Schlatter's disease (Figure 4). This anterior tibial tubercle osteochondrosis is very resistant to treatment other than rest, although orthotics do help. The mildly pronatory foot often presents a generalized postural fatigue. There is an aching felt in the posterior muscle groups. Postural fatigue is usually present only with running activity in the mildly pronated foot. This foot may also have arch fatigue and pain, as well as mild bunions and hammertoes (Figure 5). A hypermobile first ray may lead to stress fractures of adjacent metatarsals (Figures 6 and 7).

FIGURE 3
X RAY SHOWING STRESS FRACTURE OF FIBULA

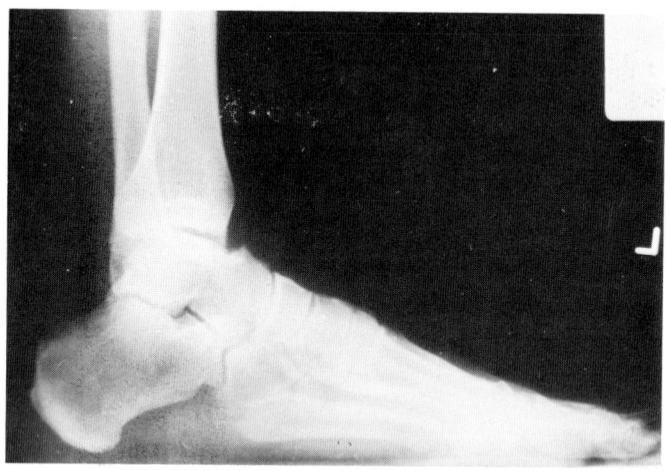

FIGURE 4
X ray Showing Osgood-Schlatter Disease

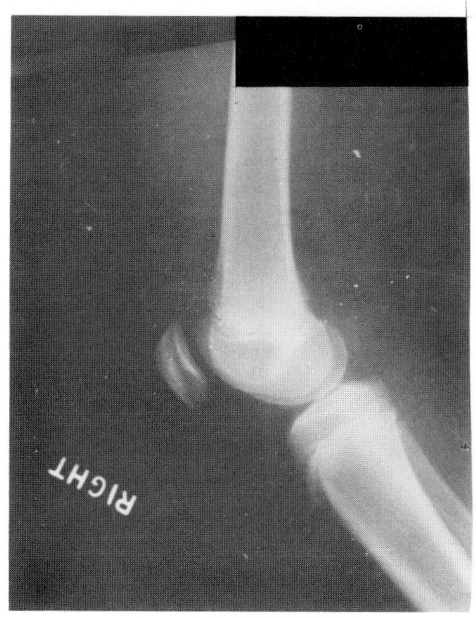

FIGURE 5
X ray Showing Morton's Foot with Stress Fracture

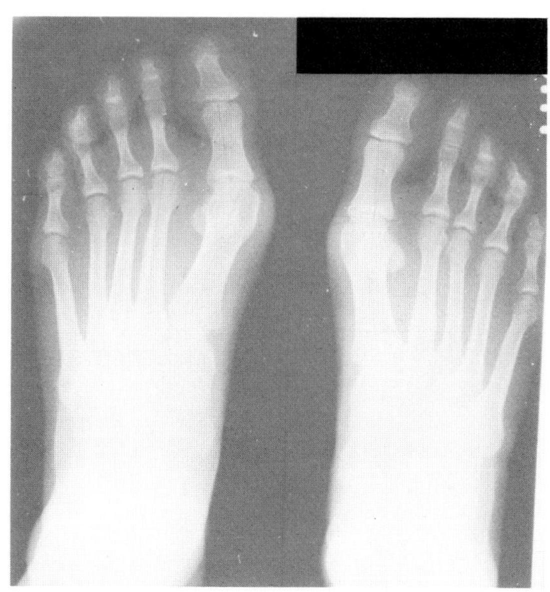

FIGURE 6
X RAY OF STRESS FRACTURE SECOND METATARSAL RIGHT

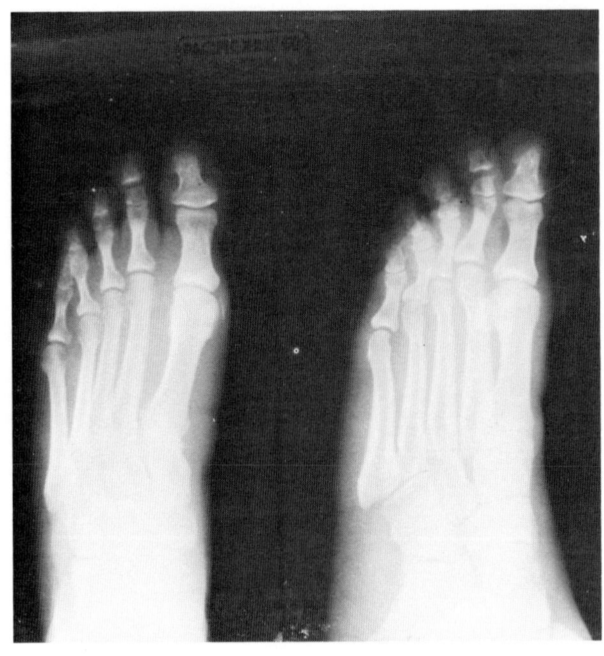

FIGURE 7A
STRESS FRACTURE SECOND METATARSAL

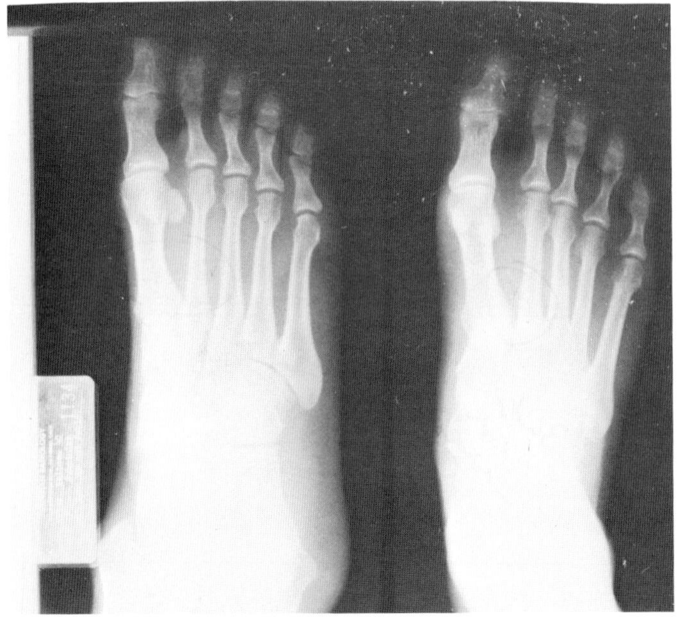

FIGURE 7B
STRESS FRACTURE 2ND METATARSAL
6 WEEKS FOLLOWING ONSET

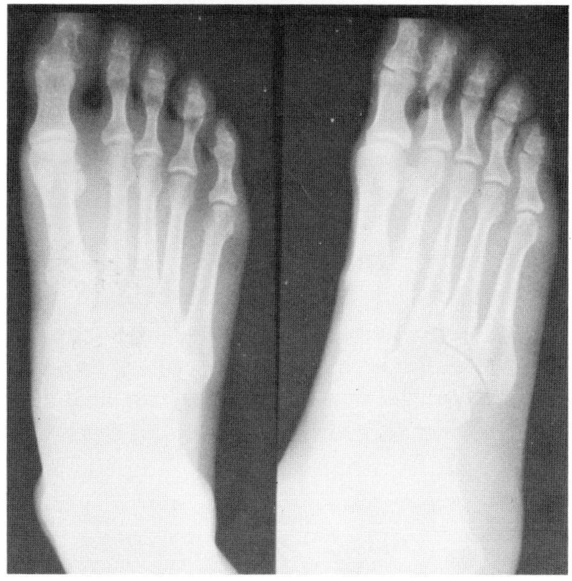

Moderately Pronated Foot

The moderately pronated foot has a calcaneal stance position of six to ten degrees of valgus (Figure 1). This also will be dependent upon the amount of tibial varum present (or internal torsion or position). Those symptoms associated with the mild calcaneal valgus are more prevalent and more severe than the moderately pronated foot. Since there is a greater amount of abnormal prolonged pronation taking place, there is greater incidence of plantar fascial strains and pulls. The intrinsic muscles of the foot fatigue sooner and the toes become unstable. These patients are more likely to have pain underneath the metatarsal heads, as well as bruises of the heel. Shin splints, chondromalacia of the knee and related patellar symptoms are more prevalent. In addition, there is a greater likelihood for collateral ligamentous strain about the knee. Plantar calcaneal spurs are more prevalent, as well as adventitious bursitis and plantar neuromas.

The range of motion of the subtalar joint appears to be somewhat increased and the midtarsal joint will generally have from six to ten degrees of forefoot varus. As the forefoot varus approaches eight degrees, it becomes more difficult to control and increased frequency of problems in the posterior flexor muscle groups, as well as increased tendencies towards tendo Achillis pull, is noticeable. The lateral compression and medial tension syndromes of the foot become prevalent with the moderate forefoot varus deformity. There may be entrapments of the nerves in the tarsal tunnel area and compression of the peroneal tendons. This runner fatigues more easily in a race and generally has a sloppy, inefficient propulsion.

If this foot is functioning maximally pronated throughout the gait cycle there is a good chance that there will be a minimal amount of swing phase resupination of the calcaneus, with the beginnings of poor shock absorbing heel contact properties. This may, in effect, cause jarring of the rest of the body with various secondary problems including stress fractures. Those deformities generally associated with the pronated foot, such as bunions, hammertoes, and fifth metatarsal head exostosis, are much more prevalent as hypermobility increases and the foot tends to splay during stance (Figure 3). Radiographically, the lateral weight-bearing view of this foot type shows incongruity of the medial longitudinal arch (Figure 8).

FIGURE 8

X RAY LATERAL WEIGHT-BEARING VIEW OF MODERATELY PRONATED FOOT

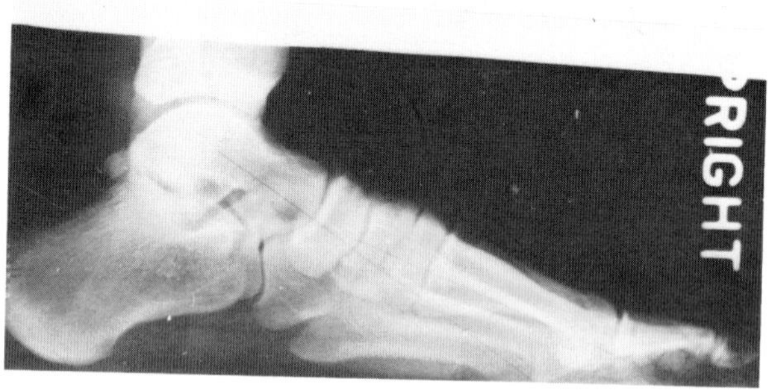

Severely Pronated Foot

The severely pronated foot generally has a calcaneal stance position of ten to fifteen degrees eversion (Figure 1). There is very little arch at all visible (Figures 9, 10, 11).[9, 11] A primary or secondary equinus deformity is present and the forefoot varus is over eight to ten degrees (Figure 12). This is the true hypermobile flatfoot, which responds only moderately well to conservative treatment. All of those symptoms associated with the moderately pronated foot are accentuated and occur frequently in the severely pronated foot. These patients have pain even without athletic endeavors and their involvement in sports makes them just that much more uncomfortable. They do respond to a semi-pronated orthotic. They will not tolerate a neutral orthotic. The aim of treatment is to control the foot just short of maximally pronated position to prevent the damage which takes place and those symptoms which take place with subluxations at the end of the range of motion. Heel lifts may be indicated. In those feet where an equinus deformity is present it may be necessary to do a tendo Achillis lengthening if all conservative treatments have failed. In those cases where tendo Achillis lengthening has been carried out, the patient could then be controlled in a neutral orthotic and many, if not all, the overuse syndromes do disappear.

FIGURE 9
X RAY SHOWING LATERAL VIEW OF PRONATED FOOT

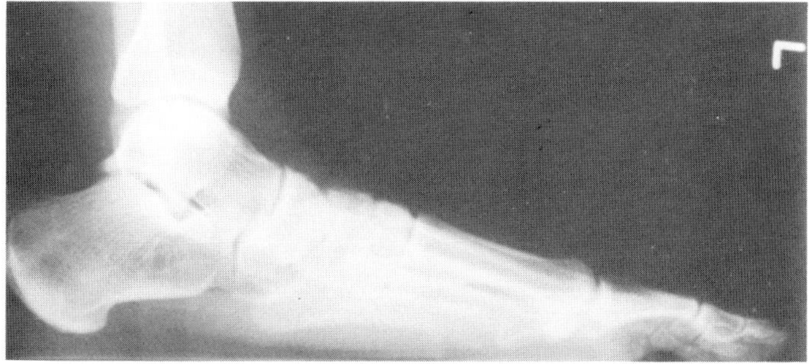

FIGURE 10
SHOWING ANTERIOR POSTERIOR VIEW OF PRONATED FOOT SECONDARY TO INTERNAL TORSION

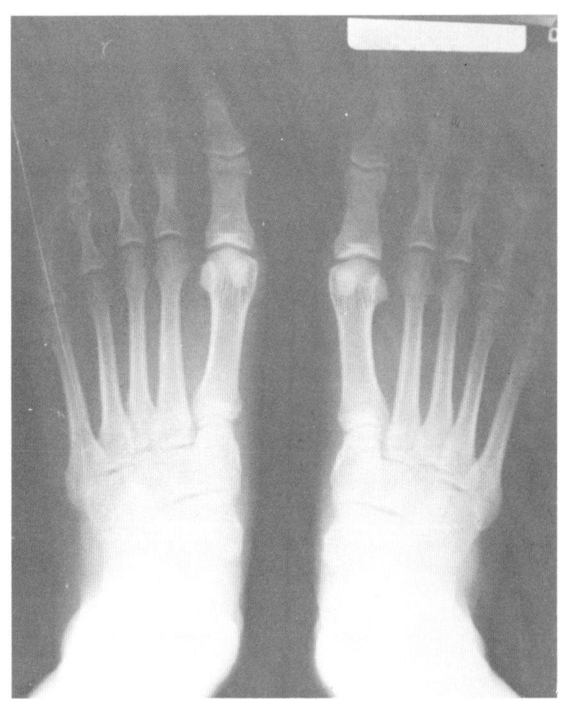

FIGURE 11
X RAY LATERAL VIEW SEVERELY PRONATED FOOT

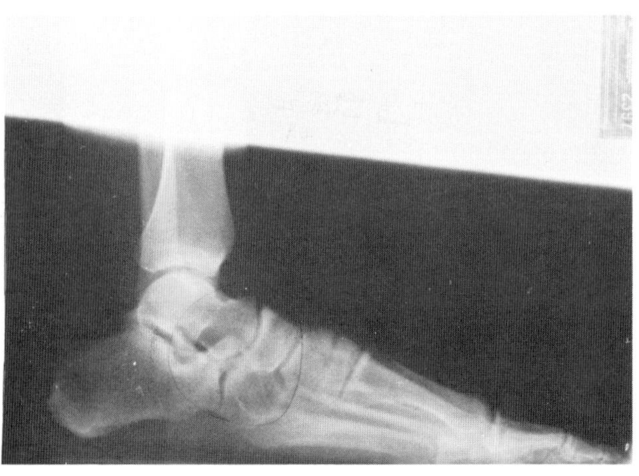

FIGURE 12

Lateral Weight Bearing X-Ray Severely Pronated Equinus Foot

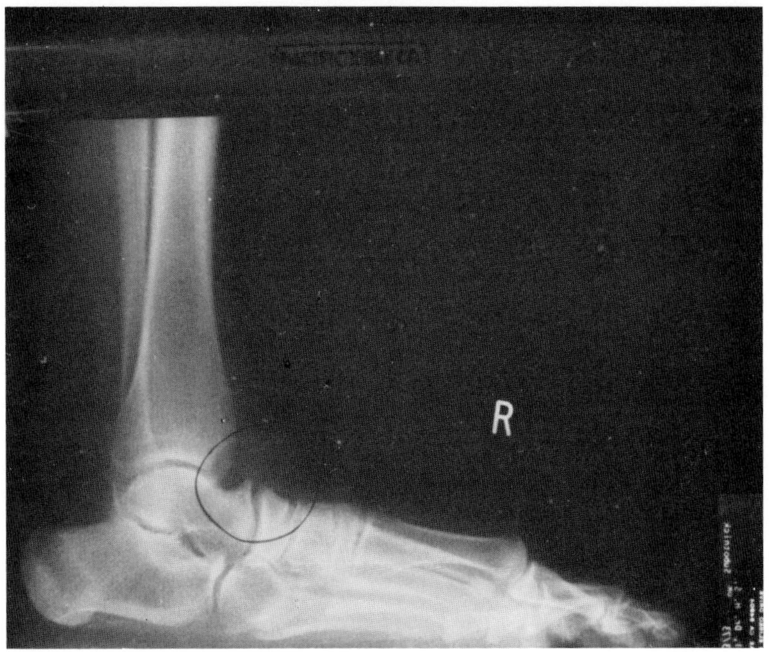

Rearfoot Varus

The rearfoot varus feet are secondary to either a varus neutral position of the subtalar joint or tibial varum (Figure 1). Both of these conditions may appear quite commonly with the forefoot varus deformity of the mild, moderate, or severely pronated foot. The rearfoot varus and tibial varum deformities are also prevalent with the various types of high arch or cavus feet (Figure 13). Those feet in which the basic deformity is rearfoot varus, however, have symptoms all of their own.

The rearfoot varus foot generally has a subtalar joint range of motion between 17 and 21 degrees, with a neutral postion of between three and five degrees varus. There may be two to five degrees of subtalar joint varus with five to seven of tibial varum in these feet. Generally, the combined rearfoot varus deformity, with subtalar joint varum and tibial varum appears to be about five to seven degrees. The subtalar joint range of pronatory motion must be used to fully or partially compensate for the rearfoot varus deformity at contact. Often times these partially compensated rearfoot varus deformities result in excessive strain upon the ankle, knee, and hip joint. This is because all of the subtalar joint pronatory motions is used up, and yet more deformities are still present and need compensation. It is easy to see how the lower extremity joints may be affected by a partially compensated rearfoot varus problem.

These feet tend to be mildly rigid and there is increased firmness of the plantar foot structures. Those symptoms present most commonly are associated with retrocalcaneal exostosis, various patellar symptoms around the knee, collateral knee strains, shin splints, plantar strains, spurs and bursae. There is also an increased tendency towards hamstring pulls, and soft tissue problems around the buttocks and hip joints. This may be due to the mild limitation of pronatory shock absorbing properties of this foot. In as much as this foot type appears to be more common in the long-distance runners, we often find these types of problems with our athletic patients in my particular office. Most of these problems have responded quite well to functional foot control.

It is usually the athletic training which results in the symptoms in this foot type. This foot type rarely causes any problems in normal day-to-day activities.

FIGURE 13
X RAY REARFOOT VARUS WITH MILD ANTERIOR EQUINUS

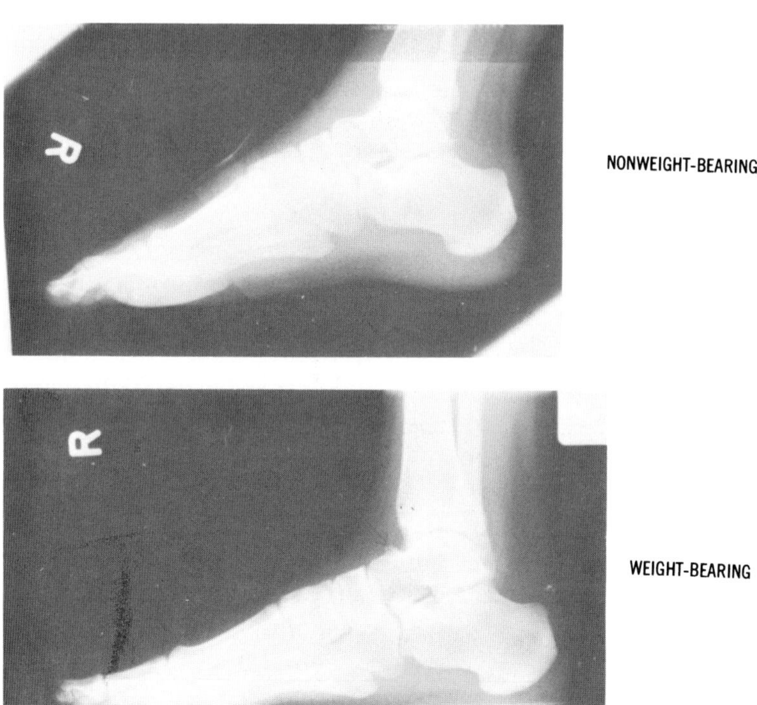

Mild Cavus Foot

The mild cavus foot has a rather high arch but the deformity is still flexible. These feet appear to have the forefoot lower than the rearfoot in what is termed an anterior equinus configuration. This high arch foot compresses somewhat on weight-bearing inasmuch as this is a dynamic deformity. The toes appear to be midly clawed in the nonweight-bearing attitude, but the clawing disappears will full weight-bearing (Figure 14). Often times the rearfoot varus is associated with this foot type. The foot is predisposed to medial calcaneal nerve entrapment, as well as plantar calcaneal bruises. In addition, the plantar fascia is often strained. The foot has somewhat limited shock absorbing properties and those problems seen with the rearfoot varus foot are accentuated in this foot type.

Initially, this foot is rather flexible and tends to accept stress somewhat better than the moderate to severe cavus foot. In time, however, this foot may progress to the more rigid cavus foot deformity, despite conservative treatment. The problem is that the time span for progression of the deformity is impossible to predict. These deformities may be idiopathic or secondary to neurological diseases (Figures 15 and 16).

The neuromuscular diseases are very difficult to diagnose and the patient may otherwise appear to be totally normal. Treatment consists of orthotics to insure proper function, as well as flexibility exercises.

FIGURE 14
X RAY LATERAL VIEW MODERATE CAVUS FOOT

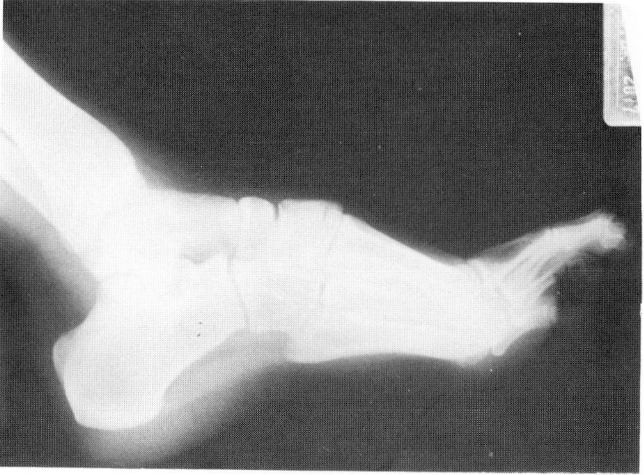

NONWEIGHT-BEARING

FIGURE 14B
WEIGHT-BEARING

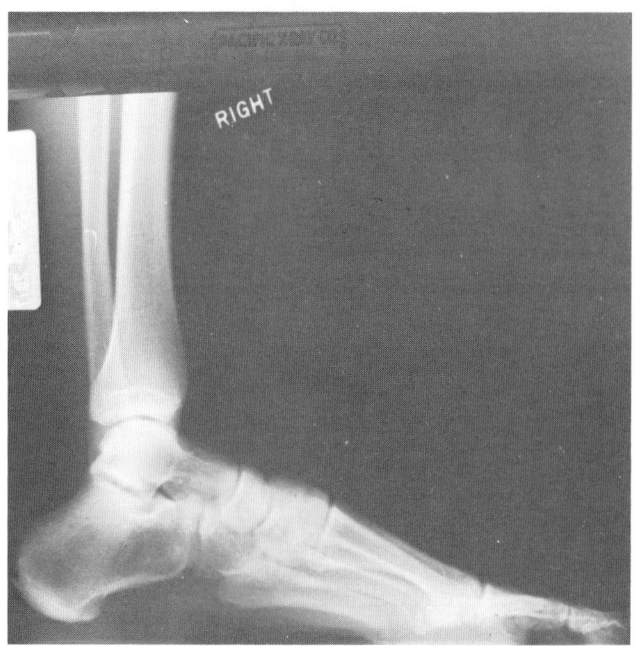

FIGURE 15
LATERAL X RAY MODERATE CAVUS WITH TALAR NECK EXOSTOSIS.

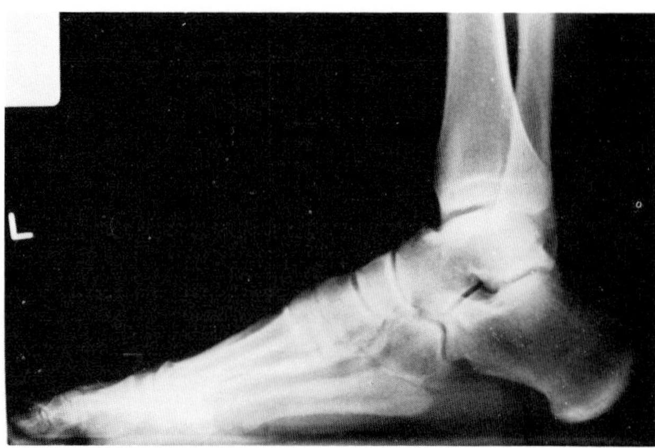

FIGURE 16
X RAY ADDUCTO-CAVUS FOOT WITH TALAR NECK EXOSTOSIS

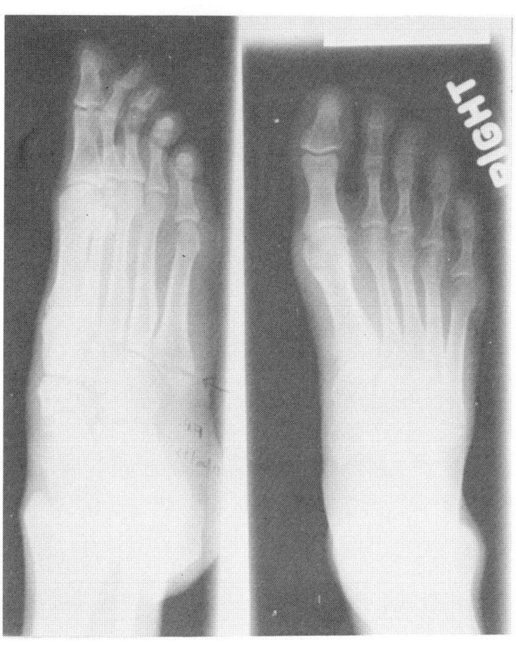

Moderate Cavus Foot

The moderate cavus foot is one in which the dangling foot exhibits claw toes which do not entirely disappear upon weight-bearing (Figure 14). This is a high arch foot which is less flexible than the mild cavus foot and which has the arch flattened only mildy upon weight bearing. The subtalar joint range of motion ranges between seventeen to twenty degrees and there is a rearfoot varus between three to five degrees. A forefoot valgus of about five degrees is normally present. The neutral calcaneal stance position is around the perpendicular. Ankle joint dorsiflexion is from eight to ten degrees. This foot has poor contact shock absorbing properties and this results in unusual forces being transmitted to the ankle, knee, thigh, buttock and back. These forces may result in injury at these levels. There is an increased tendency for sprains of the ankle with lateral collateral ligamentous damage. The knees tend to have lateral collateral strains and sometimes medial compression problems. The hamstrings are frequently injured and there may be problems around the ischial tuberosity at the origin of these muscles. There are often times low back pain and sciatica associated with this. The sciatica may also be associated with limb length discrepancy which is functional in nature and in which one foot is cavus and the other appears to be more pronated (Figure 17).

This foot is prone to having retrocalcaneal exostosis with an associated tight tendo Achillis which rubs over the exostosis (Figure 19). For this reason, there are increased pulls and strains of the tendo Achillis. The rather rigid forefoot valgus causes a great deal of pain beneath the metatarsal heads and there are generally associated intractable plantar keratomas under the more plantar directed metatarsal heads.[36] This foot tends to have a high incidence of talar exostosis secondary to impingement of the anterior talar neck upon the anterior aspect of the tibia. These talar exostosis may present pain or even go so far as to compress nerves and vessels at the ankle joint level (Figures 15, 16, 18). Stress fractures of the tibia may occur (Figure 19).

When the hammertoe deformities, as well as plantar callouses are severe enough to prevent pain-free athletic competition, surgical intervention must be considered. This intervention should be planned to slow down or impede the progression of this semi-flexible deformity to that of a rigid deformity. When symptoms are less severe, a rigid functional orthotic with a forefoot post may be utilized to help stretch out the plantar foot structures as a possible preventive measure which may slow down the progression of the foot deformity. This treatment also works rather well to control the overuse syndromes associated with this foot type.

FIGURE 17

X RAY LATERALVIEW FOOT WITH ANTERIOR EQUINUS AND RETRO-CALCANEAL EXOSTOSIS

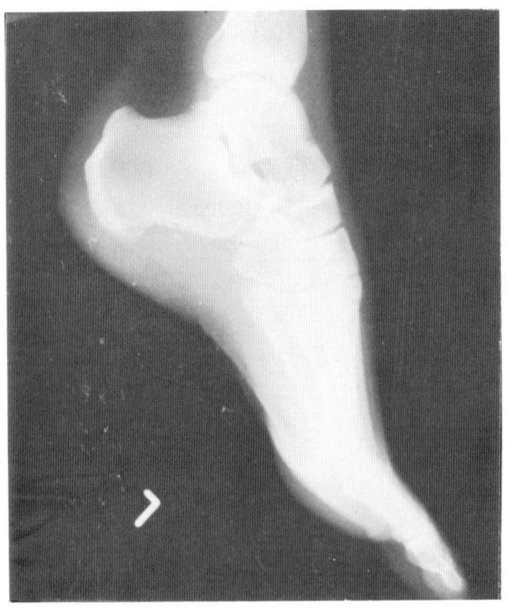

FIGURE 18
LATERAL X RAY SEVERE CATUS WITH ANKLE EQUINUS

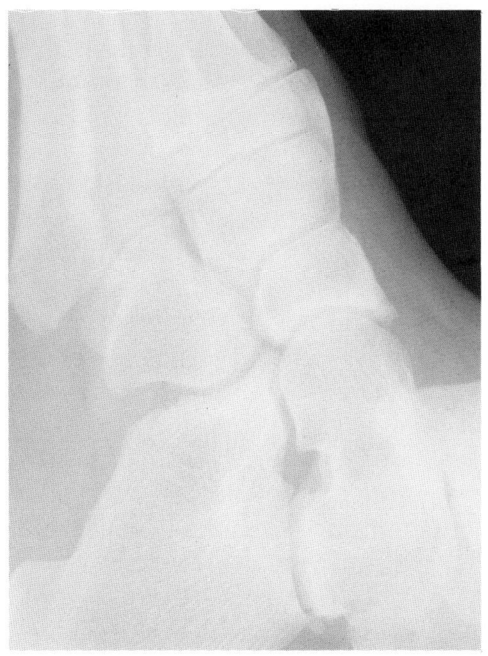

FIGURE 19
X RAY STRESS FRACTURE TIBIA

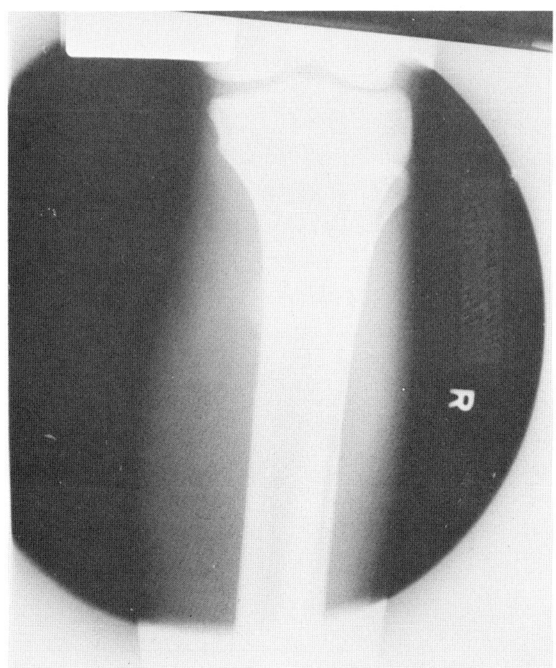

Severe Cavus Deformity

The severe cavus foot deformity is one in which the calcaneus cannot be pronated beyond a perpendicular position (Figure 17). The calcaneal stance position is usually around three to five degrees inverted. This foot has a very narrow subtalar joint range of motion and a forefoot valgus rigid deformity is often present. There are generally associated arthritic changes occurring at the midtarsal joint as well as dorsal breaking at the talar navicular joint. Talar neck dorsal exostosis are very prevalent. Clawing of all toes which do not reduce at all upon weight bearing is present. Very painful intractable plantar keratomas underneath metatarsal heads create a great deal of disability. The plantar fat pad moves anteriorally so that there is no padding beneath the metatarsal heads. The tendency towards sprained ankles is markedly increased. This foot type is poorly suited for athletic endeavors and usually requires some form of surgical intervention.

The treatment plan for the mild to moderate cavus foot deformity is to prevent progression to the more rigid cavus type foot. The nonsurgical treatment of the severe cavus foot deformity consists in utilizing various accommodative foot supports, as well as selective surgical procedures for intractable plantar keratomas and claw toes. More radical surgical procedures to correct this deformity may well be indicated. These include calcaneal and metatarsal osteotomies along with various tendon releases, transfers and transpositings.[26]

Foot Deformities Secondary to Trauma

Foot deformities secondary to trauma, usually fractures, often are in need of special accommodative supports or imaginative surgical procedures to provide for pain-free athletic function. Included in this category are fractured ankles, as well as fractured first metatarsal phalangeal joints. Traumatic arthritic joints within the foot secondary to injury or previous operations present special problems which need individual approaches to allow these patients to continue with athletic activities (Figure 20).

FIGURE 20
X ray Ankle Arthritis Following Boot Top Fracture

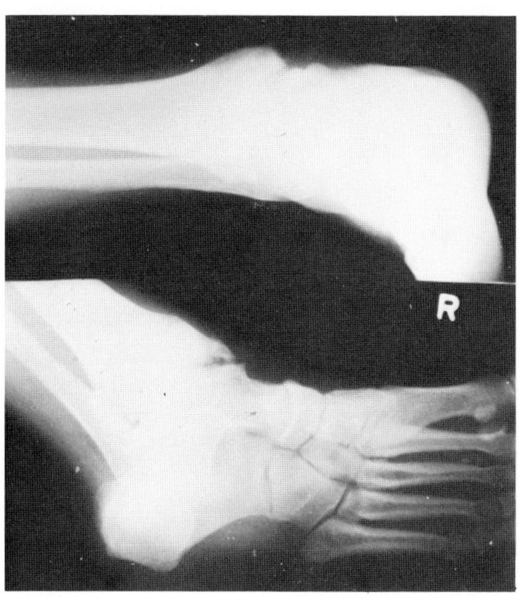

SUMMARY

In conclusion, generalizatons of symptoms associated with various foot types have been presented. These observations were gained from examining over 1,000 runners over the past four years. These are gross generalizations based more upon feelings gained, rather than strict scientific proof. The findings, however, appear to be consistent enough to warrant presenting these trends. I suggest that severe foot deformities be treated in the young athlete to help retard or prevent progression to the more rigid, less successfully treated foot types.

Chapter 8

Shin Splint Syndrome of the Lower Extremity

Shin splints is a feeling of tightness and aching which occurs during or after running and may be in either the anterior or posterior muscle group. In both cases the pain is secondary to abnormal stress upon the soft tissue structures. The muscle itself may be under strain or stress as well as the attachments of the muscle to bone, in which case a periostitis is present. Most often there is a tendonitis, myositis, and periostitis taking place. The shin splint problems of the anterior muscle groups is somewhat different from that of the posterior muscle group.

ANTERIOR MUSCLE GROUPS

The anterior muscle group includes the anterior tibial, extensor digitorum longus, and extensor hallucis longus muscle. The extensor hallucis longus is frequently associated with the shin splint syndrome. The anterior muscles are particularly prone to the shin splints type syndromes when they are overused to compensate for forefoot imbalance or a very hard heel contact. The muscle tissue becomes damaged and edema occurs. There is no place for the edema to exit because the anterior chamber of the leg is essentially a closed space. Overuse or overstrain damage to the anterior muscles may lead to a compartment syndrome. (See Appendix 1).

The anterior muscles may be overstressed or overstrained during the contact portion of gait on hard surfaces, expecially with overstriding. Forceful contact on hard surfaces may cause the anterior muscle groups to contact to aid in the deceleration of the foot as it contacts the ground. Thus, the jarring effect of heel contact during the time the anterior tibial muscles are contracting may cause excessive strain, stress, or pulling.

The anterior muscle group may be further aggravated during the mid-portion of stance at which time it forcefully contracts to help prevent a foot-slapping action when excessive forefoot varus is present. Some runners have complained of anterior muscle group shin splints following blisters to the medial plantar aspect of the foot in which case a splinting action of these muscles has occurred to protect the blistered area.

The anterior muscle group phasically is active during the swing phase, toe-off and heel contact. When the muscles are active during the stance phase of gait, they are functioning out of phase and subject to increased stress, strain, and overuse. Thus, another form of overuse is the shin splint syndrome of the anterior muscle groups.

The anterior muscle group's shin splints is best treated by exercises and periods of rest. Initially, I instruct the athlete to ice massage the anterior muscle group for ten to fifteen minutes, following a light workout, and again before retiring at night. The athlete is instructed to do his workouts on soft surfaces and, if pain persists, to rest for up to one week. Neutral orthotics are utilized so that a nonphasic functioning of the muscle is prevented. Likewise, strenghtening exercises for the anterior muscle groups are carried out by utilizing a weight shoe on the foot and dorsiflexory exercises.

Often times the anterior muscle group is weaker than a very strong posterior muscle group. A dynamic imbalance may occur between the very tight posterior muscles and somewhat weakened anterior muscles which accentuates anterior muscle group overuse.

Generally, a combination of functional orthotics, icing, and exercises as well as changing the running surfaces will aid in the treatment of shin splints. It may be necessary to utilize a shoe with thick absorbing sole during the early sessions of training.

POSTERIOR COMPARTMENT SHIN SPLINT SYNDROME

The posterior compartment of the leg, the flexor compartment, includes the posterior tibial, flexor digitorum longus, and the flexor hallucis longus muscles. These muscles, phasically, are active during the stance phase of gait from just after heel contact to just prior to heel-off. When prolonged or abnormal pronation is present at heel contact, they begin phasic activity at heel contact and are predisposed to overstress injury. Thus, the hypermobile pronated foot predisposes to posterior muscle group imbalance and shin splints syndrome.

When the posterior tibial muscle is primarily involved there may be tendonitis behind the medial malleolus and myositis more proximally. This is oftentimes complicated by periostitis. The flexors may be involved separately or combined with the posterior tibial muscle.

Posterior shin splints respond initially to ice massage twice a day, combined with functional orthotics. Range of motion exercises are carried out to increase strength and flexibility.

CHRONIC SHIN SPLINT SYNDROME

Chronic shin splint syndrome may initially require an injection of a cortico-steroid mixture to soften up an advanced scar tissue formation. Cortisone is not utilized for acute injury in which case inflammation is necessary for adequate healing.

It is often necessary to take X rays of the lower extremity to rule out stress fractures which may present with the same symptoms as shin splints. When the shin splint syndrome does not respond to neutral control and exercises, serial X rays at two week intervals may reveal stress fractures or reactions of bone. I suggest no athletic participation for at least eight weeks following the onset of the fracture. There should be evidence of bony healing. This may take up to twelve weeks. Often times acute or chronic periostitis is demonstrated radiographically. Rest is required for this inflammatory problem.

SUMMARY

The shin splint syndrome has been presented as a combination of tendonitis, periostitis and myositis of the flexor group or anterior muscle groups of the leg. The diagnosis may be complicated by stress reaction of bone or fracture.

Treatment consists of biomechanical realignment of an abnormal foot function, flexibility and strength exercises, ice massage and light workouts on soft surfaces with thicker solid running shoes.

Periods of rest from eight to twelve weeks are required for stress fracture of the leg.

Chapter 9

Dynamic Muscle Imbalance (Runner's Equinus)

Runners must be aware of the fact that strengthening and endurance exercises reduce the flexibility of the runner. Long- and middle-distance running result in overdevelopment of the muscles involved with active propulsion. These are the gravity muscles in the posterior aspects of the thigh and leg. Specifically, the gastrocnemius and soleus in the leg, as well as the hamstrings in the thigh. Such overdevelopment is relative to the lack of parallel development of the strength of the anti-gravity muscles which must check the power of this posterior muscle group. Thus, dynamic imbalances exist and appear to be favored by such activities as long-distance running. A long-distance runner characteristically has a weak quadricep mechanism, as well as weak anterior muscle groups of the leg. This antigravity weakness is accompanied by a very tight posterior muscle group which results in an actual functional equinus. I call this a runner's equinus, inasmuch as this condition is normally reversible and responds quite well to planned flexibility and stretching exercises before, and even more important, after workouts. If the activity of running causes tightness of the posterior muscle, then it appears logical to us that even more concentrated stretching should take place following running. Along with this, specific exercises should be carried out to insure strength of the antigravity muscles. I utilize straight leg raises, quadricep isometric contractions, as well as other forms of exercises such as bike riding, which favors development of the antigravity muscles if toe straps are used on pedals.

Runner's equinus can be quite a problem. It results in the same clinical symptoms as an actual anatomical equinus.[32] Equinus is defined as an inability to achieve six to eight degrees of dorsiflexion of the neutral foot upon the leg when the knee joint is extended. Normally it is safe to say six to eight degrees because with some warming up of the muscle groups most runners will go from eight degrees to ten degrees with no difficulty. Ten degrees is the actual amount of dorsiflexion which is required for normal function, inasmuch as the tibia, just prior to heel-off during the mid-stance of gait, moves forward ten degrees over the talar dome at the exact time the foot has moved out of pronation into a neutral position on its way towards full resupination.[32] Failure for the posterior muscle groups to allow this ten degrees of dorsiflexion results in a compensatory pronation of the subtalar joint to unlock the midtarsal joint and allow for dorsiflexion of the forefoot upon the rearfoot about the oblique axis of the midtarsal joint. This abnormal pronation causes the problems as we note with other biomechanical deformities resulting in prolonged abnormal pronation with lack of proper resupination. Specifically, these are the overuse syndromes.[37] In addition, there seems to be a prevalence towards tendo Achillis strain and irritations secondary to inflexibility of this muscle group.

Stretching of the gastrocnemius and soleus should be done with the knee extended and foot close to neutral position. We utilize a yoga type of approach. Stretching by jerking, bobbing, or bouncing methods (as in calisthenics) invokes the stretch reflexes which actually oppose the desired stretching. When a muscle is jerked into extension, the natural reaction is for the muscle to resist the extension and thus, shorten. Dynamic exercises are jerking in nature as compared to static yoga type exercises which utilize a slow stretch. The prolonged stretch exercise invokes the inverse myotatic reflexes which help relax the muscle being stretched.[7] Stretching, therefore, should be done gradually, with no bouncing, and the athlete should lean forward with his hands dangling towards the floor for approximately thirty seconds and then straighten up. This should be repeated three to four times, after which he will note he is stretching as well as loosening up the posterior muscle groups. In addition, leaning into the wall with the knees extended, the feet neutral, also produces a gradual stretching of the posterior muscle groups. An incline board is also helpful. Various types of yoga exercises are excellent for all of the muscle groups which may be tired and sore following a workout.

Initially, there was a tendency to overreact to tightness of the hamstrings, as well as the gastrocnemius and soleus muscle groups, that was present on the examination of long-distance runners. I now have grown to appreciate the fact that this is usually just a functional problem that needs reevaluation following a thorough stretching exercise program. Varying degrees of relaxation are noted from the almost universal severe tightness, initially present. Tightness of the posterior leg muscles which are anatomic rather than a function of overuse or improper exercise limits the amount of correction the runner can tolerate when compensating for foot imbalance or pronation with orthotics. The need for reevaluation of biomechanical findings following yoga type exercises, as illustrated in this chapter, cannot be overstressed.

Chapter 10

Orthotic Foot Control for the Athlete — The Importance of Resupination

A review of the biomechanics of running suggests that foot control by the use of orthotics may prevent excessive and abnormal pronation while restoring normal resupination. Normal resupination, beginning in midstance and terminating with the foot acting as a rigid lever during toe-off appears to be a key factor in preventing overuse syndromes as well as providing for a stable efficient lift off prior to the float phase of running. Three basic classifications of foot orthotics exists and each of them have their own characteristic uses, patient tolerance, and effectiveness for various symptoms which closely parallel the amount of functional control available. As the orthotic becomes more rigid, it approaches the more ideal functional control device. Functional control provides for normal muscle actions about stable lever systems. Functional control provides for contact shock absorbing with pronation as well as mid-stance stability and propulsive thrust. The three types of orthotics are as follows: (1) various forms of soft flexible supports ranging from felt, in a running shoe [29, 39, 40] to combinations of Spenco® and surgical orthopedic splints with various felt and rubber filler and posting devices, (2) semi-flexible supports, fabricated from surgical orthopedic splints or leather, utilizing firmer rubber compounds for posting and arch filler, (3) rigid functional orthotics fabricated from a neutral balanced cast of the patient's foot.

Rigid orthotics are formed when thermal pliable plastic is pressed over the cast which is then balanced to allow for a predetermined position of the calcaneus. This type of functional control is also known as rigid control, inasmuch as the plastic appears to be much more rigid than the felt or leather type orthotics. In reality, however, the plastic orthotics do have a certain amount of spring and give in them. The plastic orthotics are further balanced by the use of dental acrylic posts at either the rearfoot or forefoot or both. In such a way, contact, midstance, and propulsive phases of gait are controlled. Various biomechanical deformities such as rearfoot varus or valgus and/or forefoot varus or valgus are balanced, utilizing posting or cast correction. Most of the rigid devices utilize a short rearfoot post allowing for a perpendicular to two or three degrees varus calcaneal position. Since the thermal pliable plastic has intrinsic strength, it is unnecessary to have filler material and these orthotics are light and fit well into the shoes. It is necessary, often times, to remove the inner sole beneath the rearfoot post in running and other athletic shoes to prevent the heel from sliding up and down. At times, also it is desirable to remove the rubber arch pads present in athletic shoes, inasmuch as they may interfere with the function of the rigid support. If the rigid support clears the rubber arch within the shoe, there is no need to remove it. The three types of orthotics have been evaluated by means of objective and subjective findings as well as utilizing motion-analyzing photography to evaluate control of abnormal pronation and effectiveness in regard to proper resupination and propulsive stability. Runners were studied on motion-analyzing films running in shoes with no control, soft orthotics, semi-rigid orthotics, and functional rigid orthotics.

EVALUATION OF IN-SHOE PADS

Commercially available rubber arch supports which come with the various running shoes and tennis shoes offer no protection from abnormal pronation.[39] They do not appear to be at all effective in controlling symptoms of the overuse type[38]. Runners had the same amount of abnormal pronation while running in shoes with or without the commercially available arch pads. Resupination was not affected. The angle of gait was not changed.

The use of felt within the heels of shoes to provide for a varus control, did not affect the angle of gait. There was, however, some stabilization of the calcaneus and moderate oversyndromes appeared to be aided by these devices. Many of the runners related that their mild knee pains responded well to the use of varus felt pads in the heels. Along these lines some complaints of posterior tibial tendonitis and myositis were lessened with felt arch pads constructed into the running shoes. It is appraent that felt, being firmer than the commercially available rubber within the shoes, is more effective. In those cases of advance shin splints and chrondromalacia of the knees the felt was of little benefit. In those cases of medial longitudinal arch pain, the long metarsal pads made of felt did appear to be of some benefit.

The felt was well-tolerated by all of the athletes and was particularly well adapted to field event shoes, as well as sprinting shoes with spikes. The felt appeared to be useful for jumpers, as well as basketball players. Felt was useful in ski boots for mild complaints.

Thus, it is felt that in the foot with symptoms secondary to abnormal pronation, the felt will be of only minimal benefits. Film analysis showed that the foot which was maximally pronated at mid-support without felt, was also maximally pronated with the felt in the shoe and thus subjected to an inefficient toe-off in hypermobile states. It was noted that the varus heel pad did relatively little to prevent abnormal internal rotation of the leg upon the foot in regard to closed kinetic chain pronation at mid-support. The study further led one to believe that the failure of felt within an athletic shoe to prevent overuse syndromes does not correspond to the relief available by using a more rigid neutral functional control. The difference in control is considerable and control appears to be the most important factor in preventing these overuse states.

EVALUATION OF SOFT ORTHOTICS

The use of surgical orthopedic splints to fabricate a soft orthotic utilizing various forms of soft rubber and felt for posting, filler, and shock absorbing, was next evaluated. The soft orthotics were somewhat more effective than the various modifications made within the shoes themselves. They have the advantage of being readily transferred from shoe to shoe. They also have the advantage of providing increased shock absorbence as well as accommodation for painful plantar foot lesions. These devices were well-tolerated by all of the athletes and were especially adaptable to spikes as well as field event shoes. The runners related that they generally felt better with these supports and had less generalized foot symptoms when utilizing them. As the amount of control available from the support was lessened due to felt compression, symptoms tended to recur.

Review of motion-analyzing films revealed that the angle of gait was not affected and that abnormal pronation as well as normal resupination were again not affected. This suggests that the soft supports are useful for the mild to moderate overuse problems and that they may be used in combinations with functional control. Athletes should have a soft support for special events, such as sprinting and jumping and utilize a rigid functional control for everyday walking as well as distance training. Field hockey and football players appear to get better controls with the functional supports, although sprinters definitely do better with the soft flexible orthotics.

SEMI-RIGID ORTHOTICS

The semi-rigid orthotics are fabricated from a cast of the patient's foot and utilize leather as well as firm rubber cork compounds for filler and posting. These orthotics do work well for moderate overuse syndromes subjectively and objectively. They have the advantages of being fairly well-tolerated by most athletes. They have a disadvantage in that they utilize filler material for support and therefore provide for excessive bulk within the athletic shoe. In addition, the posting material does not provide the contact control available with the rigid support utilizing dental acrylic posts. Thus, it is found that the semi-rigid supports will not provide the finite control necessary for those overuse syndromes which are nonresponsive to anything but total neutral control.

It has been found that some patients with chondromalacia of the knees, not having good results with a semi-rigid support, will have excellent results with the functional plastic supports. This same principle holds true for other problems of the lower extremity.

The angle of gait is somewhat changed with the semi-rigid support depending upon the amount of bulk present in the orthotic and the position in which the major joints in the foot are held. Likewise, the toe-off may be more stable. It is felt that extremes of motion beyond the normal may be prevented with a semi-rigid support. The semi-rigid devices may be modified to provide for excellent accommodation.

EVALUATION OF FUNCTIONAL ORTHOTICS

The functional Rohadur® orthotics are fabricated from a balanced positive cast of the patient's foot. The negative impression is taken with the subtalar and midtarsal joints neutral. Structural midtarsal joint abnormalities are corrected by forefoot balancing of the positive cast. Rearfoot varus or valgus abnormalities are controlled by posting the finished orthotic. At times, both the forefoot and rearfoot posts are utilized, but by and large the majority of patients have only rearfoot posts with forefoot problems corrected by build-ups on the positive casts behind the metatarsal heads.

The functional orthotics allow for the most satisfactory control of those symptoms associated with overuse. The orthotics are well tolerated by almost all patients. They take from two to six weeks to be fully tolerated. If blisters develop, their formation is lessened by utilizing Spenco over the tops of the orthotics. The plastic orthotics extend from the heel to behind the metatarsal heads and do not interfere with toe-off. They do provide for a very stable heel contact and foot midstance. Motion-analyzing films revealed that the posted rearfoot controlled contact and did prevent abnormal pronation. Pronation does, however, occur as the foot adapts to various surface changes, yet pronation beyond the normal range of motion is eliminated. The striking feature is that even though the foot is maximally or close to maximally pronated at the beginning of midstance, resupination occurs sequentially at the desired time period during midstance and provides for a very powerful and stable toe-off during propulsion. The angle of gait is markedly changed in those athletes who have abduction of the foot secondary to abnormal pronation. The importance of a normal resupinative period during running was well appreciated by visualizing the motion-analyzing films of runners with the functional orthotics. The functional orthotics markedly affected the transverse plane rotation of the lower extremity. It is possible that flexed knee function may allow for orthotics to cause internal tibial rotation and open kinetic chain foot abduction prior to contact. This increases patellar stability.

Almost all of the athletes with kinetic functional orthotics were well pleased with them and reported that after the break-in period, they generally felt better with them than without them in both everyday and athletic shoes.

It is explained to all runners that the orthotics are not in any way a crutch which will weaken the foot. The functional orthotics allow for the joints to be moved into the proper positions by the muscles of the lower extremity to provide for proper foot function. Thus, the tendons and muscle are working around properly orientated lever systems. Orthotics used in this manner provide for proper anatomical function. The orthotics, however, are not a substitute for proper conditioning, training, and strength and flexibility. It was found that runners with very good functional control still had problems secondarily by abusing the principles of training and conditioning[38].

SUMMARY

It appears as though felt or rubber within a runner's shoe may give some indication as to the anticipated success of more sophisticated orthotics. However, it should be stressed that failure of felt or even soft orthotics does not necessarily mean that functional orthotics will not work; the difference in control is considerable. Soft orthotics appear to be useful in sprinters' shoes as well as those field event shoes which are subjected to jumping stress. Soft orthotics also are useful in ski boots which will not accept other forms of orthotics. Football and basketball shoes appear to well accept a semi-rigid or rigid orthotic. It is important to guard against too much control from which a supinatory sprain could occur. Modifications of a soft support may be useful for various dancers suffering from overuse syndromes. The rigid functional controls appear to have a definite place in the prevention of overuse injuries. They are useful for joggers, runners, and athletes such as hockey players or football players who are suffering from overuse syndromes. They are generally well accepted by all athletes but do need modification during the break-in period. Blistering appears to be the major problem which occurs during the initial break-in phases. Despite the type of orthotic which may be used during actual competition, the functional orthotics appear to be very beneficial for normal activities such as walking and standing. It has been noted that they will allow the foot to assume a proper functioning position and that the foot can hold this position for upwards to one hour even with no orthotic in the shoe. Following this period the soft tissue of the lower extremity fatigues and symptoms occur. The various forms of orthotics available have been evaluated and it is hoped that this evaluation will help you select the proper form of control for your patients.

Chapter 11

The Abuses of Orthotics in Sports Medicine

INTRODUCTION

By now, most of us are aware of some basic facts about the interrelationship between improper foot functioning and a myriad of overuse syndromes ranging from achilles tendonitis to runner's knee.[29] We appreciate that the compensated forefoot varus deformity, *Morton's Foot,* [35] leads to knee, leg, and foot symptoms. When the first metatarsal is hypermobile, abnormal pronation and lowering of the arch occurs. Chronic pronation, beyond normal limits, leads to overuse syndromes and runner's breakdown due to injury. A pronating foot is one which, as the arch is being lowered, with the foot on the ground, allows for the leg to internally rotate. This, abnormal pronation can lead to abnormal function at any level. The concept of foot supports and orthotics to counteract abnormal excessive pronation has been introduced.[38] The importance of resupination is emphasized. In this chapter we will concentrate on the misuse of orthotics.

THE MISUSE OF ORTHOTICS

Point #1

Functional orthotics are made from a *neutral* cast of the athlete's foot. This neutral cast is made with the foot in a neutral position. The neutral position is usually with the bisection of the heel parallel to the bisection of the lower one-third of the leg. In many instances, this is with the heel perpendicular to the ground. An acrylic plastic is heated and then pressed over the balanced (neutral) mold of the foot. An improperly taken cast leads to an improper mold and thus an improper orthotic. The result -- a disillusioned patient and doctor. Neutral casts, with the major foot joints in their neutral position, are hard to take. When in doubt, the doctor should always err in the direction of pronation. In other words, it is better to have the arch a bit too low rather than a bit too high on an orthotic. An orthotic that is somewhat pronated from the ideal neutral position usually results in an improved patient and never injures a runner. A cast taken with the error in the direction of supination (with the arch too high) will result in a dissatisfied and often disabled patient. As far as orthotics are concerned, too little is better than too much.

Point #2

Not all runners should have neutral control or neutral orthotics. Why? Despite a good try at flexibility exercises, there are many runners who have anatomically short hamstrings and gastrocnemius muscles. These runners with tight posterior muscular structures demand additional foot pronation beyond the ideal neutral position. Preventing this compensatory pronation results in pain taking place within the foot as well as in joints outside of the foot. Characteristically, the patient just will not tolerate the neutral orthotic and develops pain in the arch, ankle and knee. For these people, therefore, a semi-pronated functional orthotic is the answer. Heel lifts may also be indicated. Equinus refractory to pronated control and heel lifts may indicate the need for a tendo Achillis lengthening procedure. I have resorted to this procedure with good results in selected cases.

Point #3

The rigid functional orthotics should have a rearfoot post to control heel contact. However, heel contact to be biomechanically correct must allow for four to six degrees of pronation. If too much rearfoot post is used, preventing the normal pronation from taking place, a jarring heel contact will take place and there will be pain in the ankles as well as the knees. The point being that too much rearfoot post is worse than no rearfoot post. The real answer lies in having just the right amount of rearfoot post. This point of the rearfoot post providing heel contact stability is one of the major advantages of the plastic rigid orthotic over less rigid softer orthotics which, by the nature of the material, will not allow for a functional rearfoot post.

Point #4

All plastic (functional) orthotics need adjustments or minor corrections from time to time. One of the major problems in breaking in plastic appliances is the blistering which may occur on the longitudinal arch. The blistering can be lessened by adjusting the orthotics with minor lowering of the arch, as well as placing various materials over the plastic once adjustments have been made. Patients who refuse to go through the break-in and adjustments are in effect robbing themselves and the doctor of a probable favorable result. Some of our failures have come from patients who are from out of town and receive all of their treatment in one day and then have their orthotics sent to them. Although this type of treatment is sometimes unavoidable, all attempts should be made to have follow-up adjustments of the orthotics by a doctor in the area where the patient lives.

Point #5

The rigid orthotics were designed to be used in street shoes for everyday use and in training shoes or competiton shoes for long-distance work. In reality the distance is not the main point, the main point is the speed. Some runners are on their toes at a 5 ½-minute mile pace, and some at a 6-minute mile pace. The point is many runners need a more flexible, softer orthotic for faster speeds and competition. Almost all field events call for a more flexible support. The rigid support was designed for the heel-foot-toe, or the foot-toe type of gait found in jogging and long-distance running. Therefore, I find it advantageous for all athletic patients to have two pairs of orthotics. The soft orthotic is dispensed first and helps get the patient ready for the more rigid orthotic. And then the soft orthotic is used for competition, field events, and very rough cross-country courses. The rigid orthotics are used in street shoes and for training at long slow distances.

Point #6

Not all running problems are foot-related. Back pain can certainly have its origin in the back. The same with pain at any level of the body. The best orthotics in the world can't correct metabolic diseases or compensate for the abuses of proper training or conditioning principles.

SUMMARY

All devices have their uses and abuses. Understanding the abuses of orthotics helps us to better appreciate their uses. I suggest a re-evaluation of your biomechanical findings if progress is lagging. The results may surprise you and the answer to poor results may be readily apparent.

Chapter 12

The Field Treatment of Athletic Overuse Injuries (First Aid)

INTRODUCTION

Athletic injuries are secondary to two basic causes. The first cause is that of direct trauma such as a violent force, causing injury to soft tissue and/or bone. An example of this is a clipping injury in football resulting in various degrees of damage to the knee. Another example of a violent traumatic injury is the inversion sprain.

The second type of injuries in athletics are those of the overuse syndrome. The overuse syndrome is a gradual accumulation of microtraumas resulting in, at first, minor injuries which become progressively more severe. The overuse syndrome is usually secondary to a combination of three factors: (1) conditioning, (2) training, (3) biomechanical structure of the lower extremity. Thus, overuse injuries may be a combination of overtraining plus feet and legs that have intrinsic or extrinsic imbalance problems. The intrinsic deformities are those which are in the foot structure itself. Extrinsic deformities occur where a bend in the legs places the feet at an improper angle to the running surface. Imbalanced feet can result in pain in the feet, ankle, leg, knee, hip or at times, the back.[3, 5, 25, 29, 37]

Since the feet contact the running surface and support the whole body weight during running, it is not surprising that even modest imbalance, which might cause little or no discomfort during normal daily activities, can cause serious disability to the jogger, runner, or sprinter. Those athletic endeavors which utilize various forms of running are likewise affected. These problems range from stress fractures of the metatarsals to heel spurs, from shin splints to achilles tendonitis, from runners knee to sciatica syndromes. At times the use of felt and other materials inside a well-constructed running shoe will correct minimal imbalances and those symptoms associated will lessen. At other times, the overuse pain will be decreased, but is still bothersome.

Felt, therefore, may help a runner through a race as well as give an indication that the pain being experienced may be secondary to an improper foot functioning.

Failure of felt or other materials such as rubber being utilized in an athletic shoe does not mean that a well-made orthotic, fashioned from a neutral cast of the athlete's foot, will also fail. The difference in control available with felt and other similar materials as compared to the more rigid orthotics is considerable.

When such simple measures as utilizing felt within an athletic shoe fail, then a permanent orthotic should be constructed for balancing and control. When the podiatrist feels that the feet in themselves are not the primary cause of the athletic pain, a thorough assessment of the muscular systems may reveal the etiology. Muscular balance, strength, and flexibility must be evaluated. Short or tight gastrocnemius and hamstrings should particularly be evaluated in cases of recurrent strains. Likewise, weak quadriceps and medial hamstrings with patellar problems.

The following are guides for the use of various readily available materials in the treatment of an athletic: felt, moleskin, and tape are available from surgical supply houses. Most podiatrists have these materials on hand at all times. Various shaped rubber wedges are likewise available from medical and podiatry supply houses. Polyurethane is available in various thicknesses from furniture factories. There are usually sufficient scraps available at no charge to meet the needs of both the athlete and the sports medicine podiatrist.

MOLESKIN

Moleskin is available with adherent and is utilized to lessen or to prevent blistering under metatarsal heads or bony prominences of the feet. Many runners prefer to use moleskin on the bottoms of their feet, yet tape their toes over bony prominences to prevent blistering. Moleskin may be used around the malleoli in cases of friction damage to the skin in ski boots, ice skates, or other similar foot gear.

Many athletes will attempt to use moleskin to lessen the symptoms of callouses on the plantar surfaces of the feet. This form of treatment has met with various degrees of success which are usually only temporary due to the fact that improper functioning of the metatarsal heads is the primary cause of callouses in the forefoot area. The formation of the so-called intractable plantar keratomas is secondary to the shearing forces of metatarsal heads rolling over the skin. The definitive treatment for this problem is a well-constructed orthotic which prevents this abnormal metatarsal head motion.

SPENCO ®[1]

Spenco and related substances are specifically designed to reduce shearing forces and absorb shock. Spenco is a type of rubber impregnated by nitrogen. Many running shoes have spenco insoles already in them. Spenco is available in most sporting good stores and sports medicine specialists usually have Spenco on hand in their offices. We utilize Spenco over the tops of rigid orthotics to decrease the likelihood of blister formation during the break-in period. Spenco is also useful for those sports and activities where jumping is present to reduce the shock of heel contact. Many long-distance runners do like Spenco over their orthotics used for training.

POLYURETHANE

Polyurethane is very helpful in the treatment of heel bruises and spurs. Various thicknesses of the polyurethane ranging from ½ inch up to 2 inches are utilized to fabricate a heel pad. The center of this pad may be hollowed out to accomodate the bruised area of the plantar aspect of the heel. When this is placed in the athletic shoe it helps with the symptoms associated with the painful heel. The thinner sheets of polyurethane are useful in the forefoot aspect of the shoe to lessen the shock of foot contact when running on harder surfaces. This may be helpful in lessening or preventing the shin splints syndromes of the anterior muscle groups. The anterior muscle groups decelerate the foot during contact and we have found that the polyurethane cushions the blow of the forefoot coming to the running surface and decreases the strain upon the anterior muscle groups.

MOLDABLE PODIATRIC COMPOUND ®[2]

Moldable podiatric compound is available from General Electric Corporation and is utilized to fabricate various ortho-digital devices. This material may be molded between and around toes to help support them and straighten them. Thus we have found useful to make ortho-digital devices for the chronic strains of the long flexors of the toes. In addition, this material is excellent for soft corns between toes.

[1] Spenco Trademark

[2] General Electric Company

ONE-QUARTER INCH HEEL PADS

One-quarter inch heel pads are made out of surgical felt.[29, 35, 39, 40] Surgical felt is white and is available with an adherent on one side. Since most runners have some bowing of the lower one third of the legs, I have found that the use of one-quarter inch surgical felt on the inside of the heel which is tapered down so that there is no felt beyond the middle of the heel, provides for control of minor malpositions. I term this a *varus* heel pad (Figure 1). The malpositions responding to treatment with the varus heel pad occur mainly within the legs or within the subtalar joint. Those athletes with tibial varum usually notice that they are bow-legged.

FIGURE 1
One-Quarter Inch Varus Heel Felt Pad

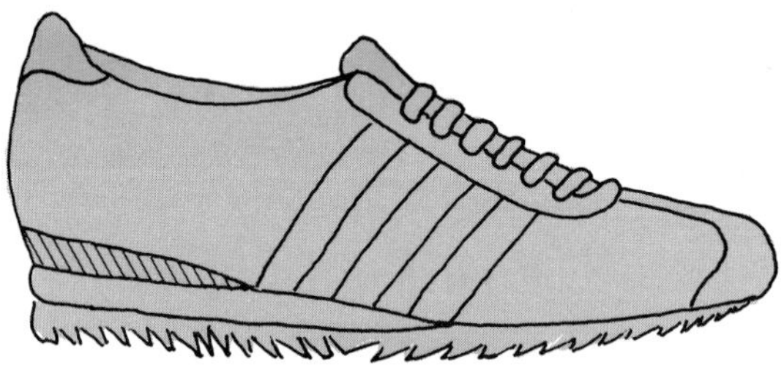

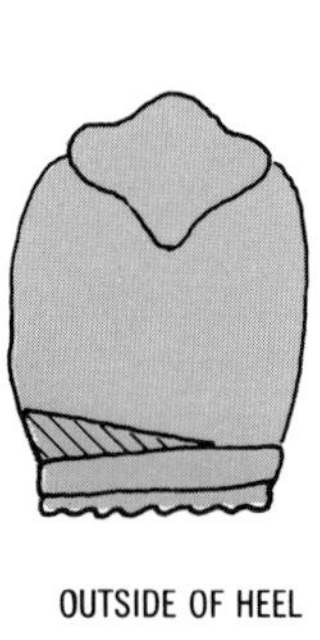

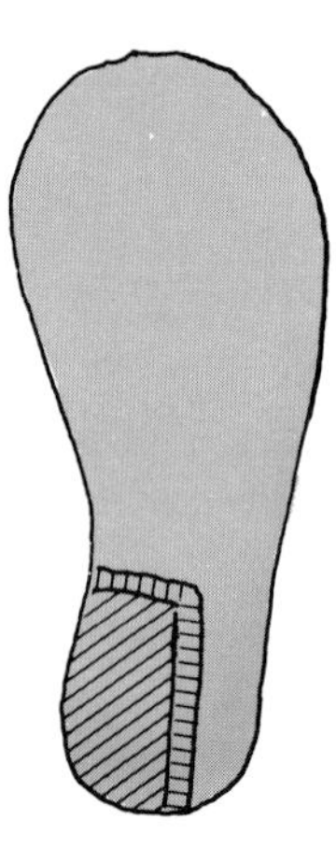

It is explained to the athlete with a subtalar joint varum that the subtalar joint functions as a universal joint beneath the ankle joint. Running and ambulation utilize various amounts of tranverse plane rotations and these are absorbed by the subtalar joint of the foot. Because the ground disallows the foot to either internally or externally rotate, the subtalar joint reflects this type of motion by either inversion or eversion of the calcaneus. This is synonymous with supination or pronation of the foot. It is important for the athlete to realize that as he lowers the arch of the foot, the leg internally rotates. As the arch is raised, the leg externally rotates. These are closed-kinetic chain reactions, inasmuch as the foot is firmly placed upon the ground. Because of this unique interrelationship between transverse plane rotations and pronation or supination of the subtalar joint of the foot, the athlete begins to realize that foot imbalance can very well lead to problems anywhere in the lower extremity proximal to the foot.

Thus, a bow-legged or varus condition will cause heel strike on the outside of the heel. The runner will be concerned with excessive wear of the shoe on the outside of the heel. Along with this unusual shoe wear, there may also be various overuse problems, such as runner's knee or retro-calcaneal irritations referred to as "runner's bumps." Shin splints are also more prevalent. Thus, we utilize the varus heel pad to help with those problems, such as runner's knee, shin splints, or "runner's bumps" (irritations on the outside of the heel near the attachment of the heel cord). The athlete, of course, must understand that these measures are usually temporary and that if the pain associated with the abnormal function does not completely disappear, but only lessens, then it will be necessary to have a more permanent biomechanically sound form of orthotic constructed.

A full one-quarter inch pad with the center hollowed out may be utilized for heel bruises or heel spur syndrome with various degrees of success. You may also utilize the one-quarter inch and one-eighth inch surgical felt in various combinations to help balance up lower extremities with anatomical limb length discrepancies.

ONE-QUARTER INCH SURGICAL FELT HEMI-VALENTINE PAD

An arch pad which is shaped like half of a valentine is made of one-quarter inch surgical felt. This is utilized for those overuse syndromes associated with pronation of the foot occurring mainly at the midtarsal joint. Of course, there will also be some pronation of the subtalar joint occurring. Thus, various forms of foot strain, such as plantar fasciitis, or myositis of the intrinsic foot muscles are treated with this felt pad which rests in the hollow of the arch of the foot. The pad may also help lessen the symptoms associated with muscle pulls, shin splints, and knee problems which appear to be related to a sagging of the arch. The felt arch pad is beveled in such a manner that it fits well the contour of the plantar aspect of the foot. It extends from the anterior aspect of the calcaneus to just behind the metatarsal heads. In the case of the short first metatarsal (Morton's Foot) the pad may be extended beyond the first metatarsal head for additional medial foot support. Variations of this felt pad can be utilized likewise to accommodate prominent metatarsal heads with associated callouses (Figure 2).

FIGURE 2

Felt Pad With Accommodation and Morton's Extension

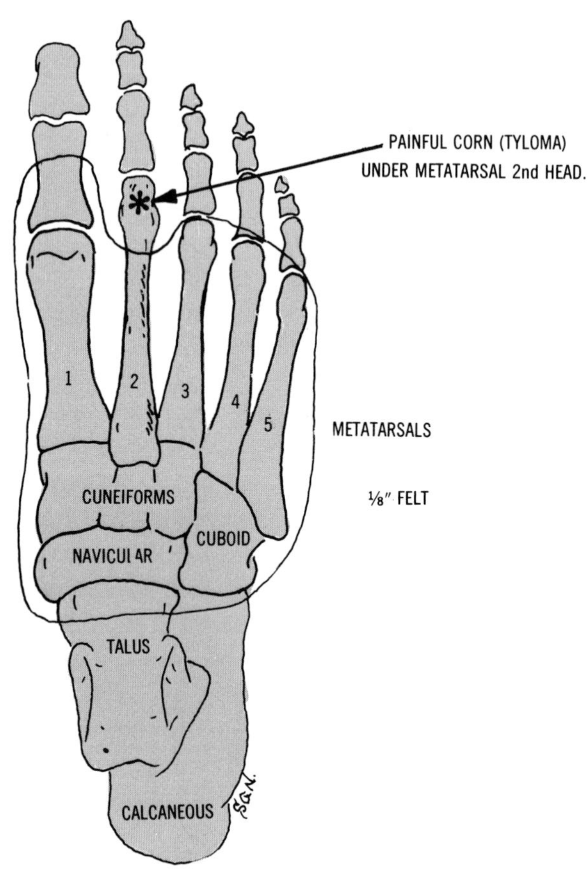

ONE-EIGHTH INCH SURGICAL FELT

One-eighth inch surgical felt has many uses. It may be used for additional padding beneath the metatarsal heads. It may be utilized to form accommodative devices to pad prominent bony spurs. It may be utilized in various athletic shoes to narrow a heel or to prevent slipping forward in the shoe by being placed underneath the tongue of the shoe (Figure 3).

FIGURE 3
FELT ARCH PAD

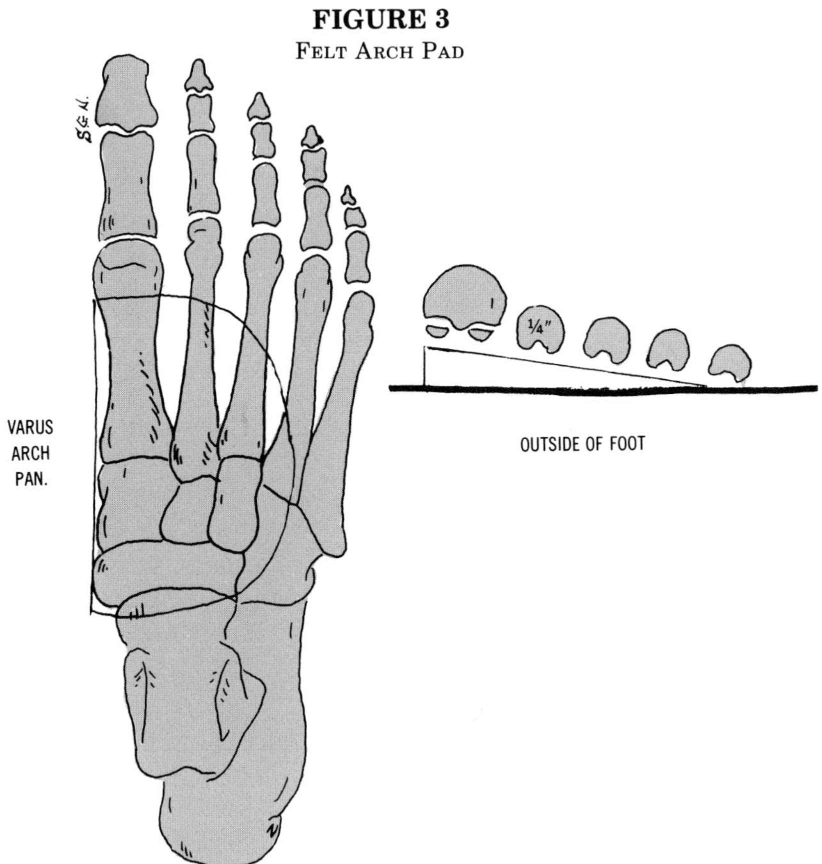

RUBBER HEEL WEDGES AND ARCH PADS

Commercially available, beveled rubber heel wedges and arch "cookies" may be applied to the inside of an athletic shoe with rubber cement. These materials are used in the same way as felt and have the same indication. They have the advantages of being more permanent than felt, yet the disadvantages of being firmer and sometimes less easily tolerated.

SUMMARY

In summation, then, various relatively inexpensive, soft materials which are well-known to the profession of podiatry have been presented with respect to their utilization in sports medicine. It is to be stressed that utilizing these materials as *first-aid* measures has varying results. They range from complete elimination of a nagging problem, which allows for competition in an athletic event, to moderate decrease in the symptoms associated with an overuse problem. Failure of these soft materials does not mean that a functional orthotic made from the neutral cast of the athlete's foot will also fail. There is a vast difference in the control available between the softer materials and the more rigid orthotics. Inasmuch as rigid orthotics are not applicable to all forms of athletic endeavor, the utilization of these soft materials is of paramount importance.

Chapter 13

The Use of Tape for Prevention and Treatment of Lower Extremity Athletic Injuries

INTRODUCTION

Athletic taping is well known to most trainers and coaches. Some professional football and basketball teams fine their players if they fail to tape their ankles prior to practicing or competing in a game. Taping definitely has a place in sports medicine. A review of anatomical considerations and biomechanical factors which influence the methods of tape application will be presented in this chapter. Properly applied tape takes on the function of a flexible cast which aids in the prevention of athletic injuries and rests injured parts to aid in their healing. This flexible tape cast limits motion. It places soft tissue parts in a semi-corrected postion, and assists in healing while providing for protection from pressure or contact. Tape, furthermore, provides for compression and may help to decrease local swelling. Tape actually acts as a form of an external ligament which prevents excessive motion beyond the normal ranges of motion. In this way, motion is really not limited but excessive motion which may be damaging to the body is prevented. By creating local traction and helping prevent further injury to a part, a good taping may eliminate the need for plaster of paris immobilization of the lower extremity for lesser injuries. Thus, we find that tape basically acts as an external splint which may rest parts, as well as prevent excessive motion.[4, 15, 18]

A rough classification of sports injuries which have proven most tractable in the use of adhesive tapes includes sprains, strains, ruptures, myositis, tendonitis, torn ligaments, fasciitis, arthralgia, fractures, small ulcers or wounds, compression on ganglion, prevention against new injuries and protection against further damage from chronic injuries. The use of tape, as well as felt, is helpful to prevent some of the minor to moderate symptoms associated with overuse and hypermobility of the foot.

APPLICATION OF TAPE

Prior to the application of tape, the skin should be well cleansed with soap and water and all hair should be removed from the area of injury. We find it useful in our practice to apply tincture of benzoin to the skin prior to the application of tape. Various forms of spray-on adherent are also useful. Various felt pads to invert or evert the heel or to compensate for forefoot varus or valgus are utilized on the foot before the tape is applied. Knowledge of the axis of motion of the various joints or the lower extremity are utilized when applying the tape.[23] An example of this would be moderately supinating the subtalar joint to rest an injured posterior tibial tendon in the case of a posterior shin splint. Thus, we attempt to invert the foot to rest a posterior muscle. We recall that open kinetic chain supination has the three motions of plantar flexion, inversion, and adduction of the foot. Open chain pronation has the motions of dorsiflexion, eversion, and abduction of the foot. Tape to stabilize the subtalar joint is applied to assure tri-plane fixation when immobilzing the heel. The subtalar joint is never totally immobilized by using tape, yet extremes of motion are prevented. In a similar manner, when one is applying tape for a hypermobile state of the foot, the midtarsal joint must be considered. A stable midtarsal joint is maximally pronated and often times a medial longitudinal arch is helpful when it is encompassed in the tape job. This is especially true for problems with the foot itself as well as those of the lower extremity related to abnormal midtarsal joint pronation.

While the subtalar joint and midtarsal joints of the foot are triplane axis joints which have motion around a pronatory-supinatory axis, the ankle joint is a hinge-type joint with some reservations. Abnormal motion occurs with excessive inversion or eversion of the calcaneus, placing concommitant abnormal strain upon the lateral and medial collateral ligaments. It is possible to limit abnormal motion at the ankle joint beyond the normal ranges of motion in regard to inversion or eversion of the calcaneus without markedly limiting dorsiflexion or plantarflexion of the foot at the ankle joint. Along these lines, tape can then protect the foot from ankle sprains while allowing for proper function on the sagittal plane. Other hinge type joints within the foot are those of the metatarsal-phalangeal and interphalangeal joints. Likewise, these joints may be stabilized while still allowing some motion on the sagittal planes, if desired.

When an injury has already occurred or the patient has a history of chronic injuries, it is best to apply the tape over the skin itself. An exception to this would be if there is an allergy to tape, in which case, tape may be applied over roller-gauze or kling. It may be necessary to use hypoallergic tape for some athletes. In cases where preventive taping is carried out and no history of injury is present it is permissible to apply the tape over a stocking. Bear in mind that tape, at best, provides a flexible type cast function, and should not be utilized when complete immobilizaton in plaster of paris is indicated. Specific considerations for taping techniques for various injuries of the lower extremity will follow.

STRAPPING TO PREVENT ANKLE SPRAINS

The collateral ligaments of the ankle joint actually cross the subtalar joint. Nonelastic tape is used to strap the ankle, since the object of strapping is to both support the ankle and reduce lateral mobility of this joint. In reducing lateral mobility, we prevent excessive pronation and supination of the subtalar joint with concommitant injury to the collateral ligaments. Following preparation of the skin, the foot and ankle are wrapped with roller gauze or kling to help reduce skin irritation (Figure 1). Two to four overlapping stirrups of 1 ½ inch tape are placed, beginning about three inches above the medial malleolus and running beneath the heel, terminating at the same level on the outside (Figure 2). Purposes of the stirrups are to prevent the ankle from abnormal amount of inversion and eversion. Tape is applied next in configuration known as the "Louisiana Heel Lock." The heel lock begins just forward of the malleolus medially and runs over the top of the instep, then beneath the arch, around the heel, over the instep agin, beneath arch, around the heel a second time, then back around the foot and terminates with a double wrap around the lower leg (Figure 3). An anchor strip is added to the top of the strapping to prevent excessive pulling of the skin (Figure 4). Care must be taken not to apply tape too tightly or circulation will be impaired resulting in a breakdown of skin. Tape is properly applied with the amount of tension needed to remove the tape from the roll.

STRAPPING THE SPRAINED ANKLE

When an ankle sprain has occurred, taping is accomplished with a nonelastic tape applied directly to the skin to provide maximum support. An open-face basket weave, utilizing horizontal saddle straps and longitudinal stirrup straps, is preferred. This basket weave is essentially a modification of the classic Gibney Ankle Strap (Figure 5,6,7). This type of strap maintains ankle support yet provides for dorsal and plantar flexion. It is, in effect, a supportive dressing for the medial and lateral collateral ligament of the ankle joint. The calcaneus is further stabalized with a heel lock. The anterior ankle capsule and tibial-tibular syndesmosis is protected with a figure of eight wrap.

PREVENTATIVE ANKLE STRAPPING

FIGURE 1
PREVENTATIVE ANKLE STRAPPING

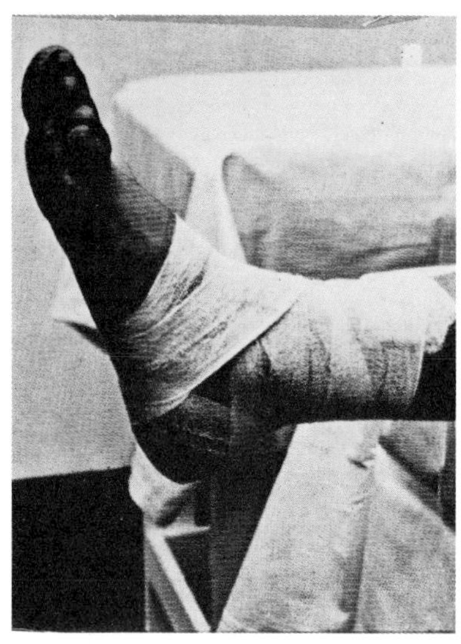

FIGURE 2
OVERLAPPING STIRRUPS-CONTROL EVERSION AND INVERSION

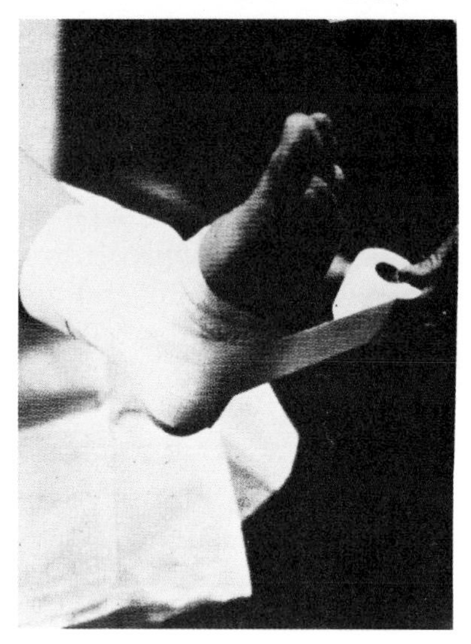

FIGURE 3
LOUISIANA HEEL LOCK

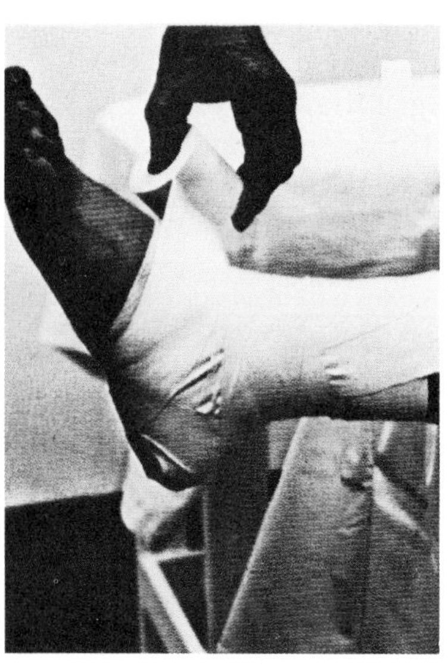

FIGURE 4
ANCHOR ADDED

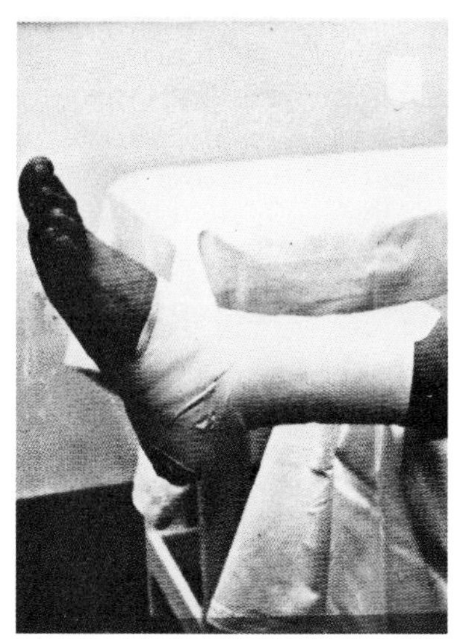

FIGURE 5
BASKET WEAVE - HORIZONTAL AND LATERAL STIRRUPS

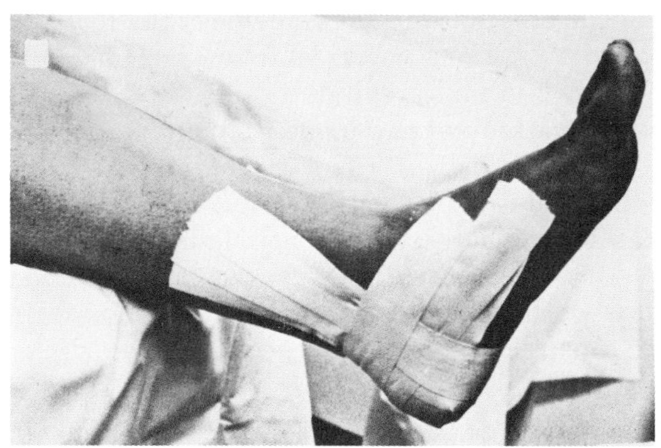

FIGURE 6
BASKET WEAVE

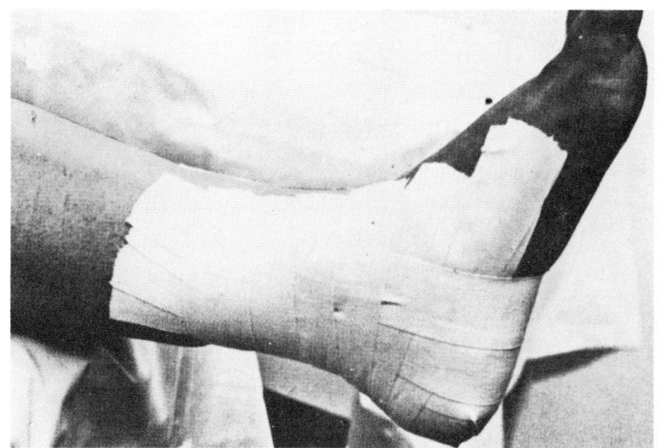

FIGURE 7
ANCHORS

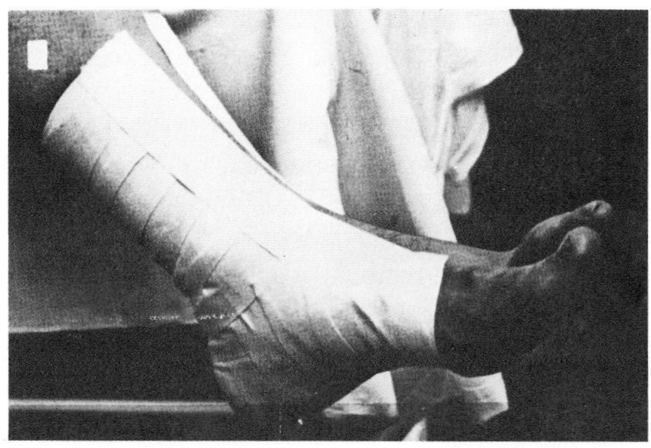

FOOT STRAPPINGS

I have found it advantageous in the treatment of overuse syndromes and chronic soft tissue problems of the foot to utilize the removable combinations of the elastic tape and felt. In cases where hypermobile midtarsal joint is present, we utilize a longitudinal felt metatarsal pad made from quarter inch scived felt which extends from just anterior to the plantar surface of the heel to behind the metatarsal heads. The felt is thicker on its medial border than lateral border. It essentially fills in the arch area of the foot. Two or three inch elastic tape is placed around the instep of the foot with the sticky side out. The felt pad is then placed in position in the arch of the foot and secured by elastic tape placed again around the instep of the foot with the sticky side down. In this manner the felt and elastic tape may be removed to allow for bathing or soaking. This type of flexible device is useful for dancers as well as athletes involved in running and contact sports. This type of device is particularly useful for plantar fascial strains as well as metatarsal problems. The felt may be extended proximally under the heel to accomodate stone bruises or adventitious bursitis and heel spurs. In these cases an aperture is cut out of the felt for accommodation. Plantar calcaneal fasciitis and bursitis are therefore treated with this soft device along with injection therapy consisting of cortico-steroids and hyaluronidase (Wydase®). Following the acute phase of the plantar heel problem, the patient is placed in a functional plastic orthotic to prevent recurrence.

Removable crest pads have been used for treatments of strain of the long toe flexors, know as *pseudo-shin splints*. Likewise, tape is often applied to toes to prevent blistering which occurs during races and long training runs.

Stress fractures of the foot, which have been allowed to heal for three weeks, may be treated for the next three weeks with a long metatarsal pad as well as a low-dye strapping (Figures 8 and 9). A variation of this type of strap consists simply of a long metatarsal pad which is secured with two to three inch tape wrapped circumferentially around the instep of the foot. The felt must be fabricated in such a way as to support the metatarsals. The classic low-dye strap is also very beneficial for acute arch symptoms.

Combinations of overuse symptoms secondary to tibial and subtalar joint varum are generally treated with felt alone within the running shoe. In the case of muscle tendon strains associated with these varus deformities, taping which rests the injured part utilizing felt and tape is beneficial. Long-term treatment of these problems is better achieved by using a functional foot orthotic (Figures 8 and 9).

FIGURE 8
LONG METATARSAL PAD

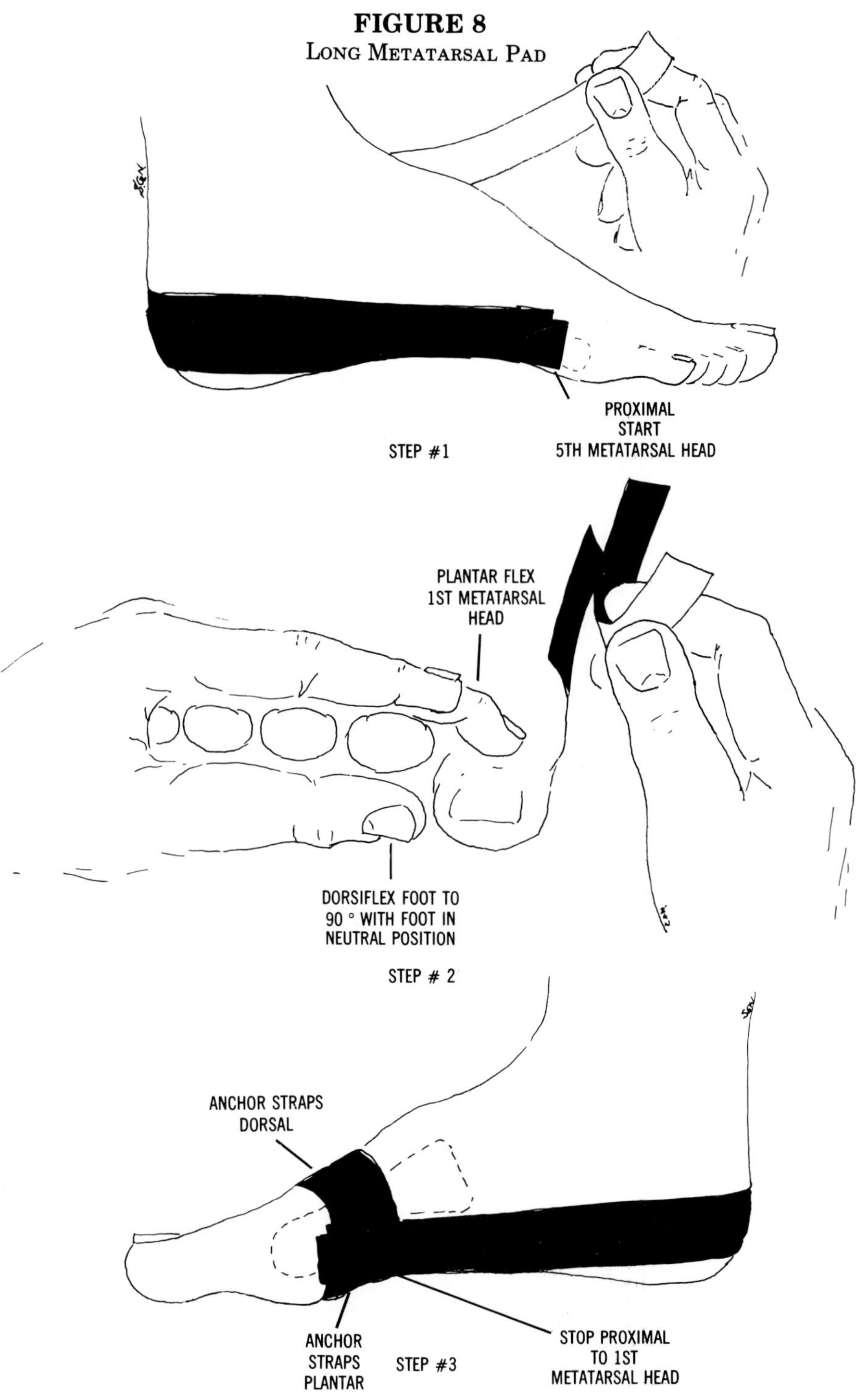

FIGURE 9
Low Dye Strapping

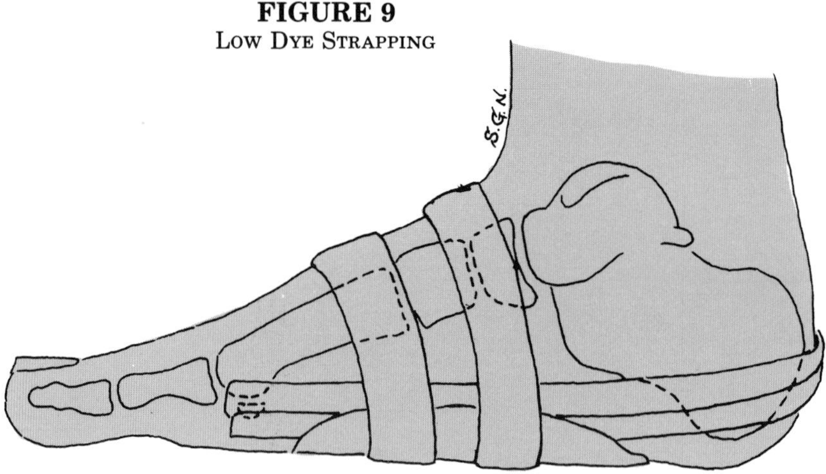

RUNNER'S KNEE (CHONDROMALACIA OF THE PATELLA)

Chondromalacia of the knee occurs secondary to abnormal patellar function which may be inherent in the functioning of the knee joint itself or secondary to abnormal foot function. In these cases, we have found it useful, along with properly prescribed exercises, to utilize foot control as well as strappings of the knee for the more acute problems. It is beneficial to use a horseshoe-shaped felt pad placed at the lateral aspect of the patella held in place with an elastic bandage, which crisscrosses the front of the knee joint.This type of wrapping helps to prevent excessive lateral subluxation of the patella during running. It also prevents excessive knee flexion which helps ease the overuse of the patella. When the symptoms become less severe, an elastic knee support may be helpful to provide compression and somewhat minimize lateral movement of the patella. These are used in conjunction with functional orthotics with a rearfoot post to minimize abnormal transverse plane rotation of the leg which might occur with abnormal closed kinetic chain pronation. This will be discussed further in Chapter 14.

LIMB LENGTH DISCREPANCIES

Limb length discrepancies with a pelvic tilt may be secondary to a true anatomical shortening, as well as a functional shortening. Likewise, the pelvic tilt may be secondary to a combination of a functional and anatomical shortening of a lower extremity. This will be discussed in greater detail in Appendix 3. Combinations of felt heel lifts, as well as felt longitudinal pads, with tape to prevent excessive pronation of the foot, help to distinguish between functional and anatomical shortenings. They also may ease symptoms associated with the low back syndrome secondary to a short limb, while the doctor and patient are waiting for more functional control devices to be fabricated. It is important to hold both feet close to a neutral position and then makeup for any difference in limb length with a heel lift. When this is carried out those symtpoms associated with sciatica and low back pain often times are lessened or will disappear.

TENDONITIS

The use of tape for the treatment of tendonitis is two-fold. Firstly, the tape provides for compression of the injured structures and secondly, it will rest the injured structure. It is necessary to place the foot near the end of the range of motion in which the tendon muscle unit pulls the foot. In this way, the unit is rested. It is often necessary to use combinations of felt and tape when carrying this out. Immediately following acute myositis or tenosynovitis, taping to provide moderate compression and relaxation of the involved motion units provides good results. When the posterior muscle groups are involved, it is often times advisable to incorporate a quarter inch heel lift into the tape job. In the case of contusions half inch foam rubber pads over the injured muscle, in combination with ace wraps, provide adequate mobilization and compression. Likewise, herniation of the various muscles can be temporarily treated with moderate compression over the part utilizing felt pads and tape. Long term problems require functional control of the foot with a rigid orthotic.

SHIN SPLINTS

Shin splints may occur in the anterior or posterior muscle groups of the lower extremity. Unless they are acute in nature, they may be treated with a combination of exercises as well as icing, and foot supports. Acute cases are treated with compression tapings which help stabilize the muscles and prevent irritation at the attachment of the muscle to bone. Thus, this minimizes the periostitis and myositis which accompanies shin splints.

SUMMARY

The use of tape as a flexible splint, has been presented. It is pointed out that it is useful as a protective device to help minimize those injuries which occur at the ends of extremes of range of motion. Tape does not prevent motion, it merely limits excessive motion. Various combinations of tape, felt, and elastic tape, have been presented and, in general, the short-term effects of these devices are most satisfactory. We suggest that in most instances, where symptoms are secondary to abnormal motions of the subtalar or metatarsal joints of the foot, the use of felt and tape is of a temporary nature and a more permanent, long-standing and functional device is necessary. This is achieved with a rigid orthotic. A thorough knowledge of various strappings is essential for the podiatrist associated with athletes, inasmuch as immediate, adequate, temporary relief for symptoms is often times accomplished with these modalities.

Chapter 14

Chondromalacia of the Knee and Related Conditions

Chondromalacia of the knee (runner's knee) and related conditions are commonly encountered in joggers and long-distance runners.[24] A variation of this problem is known as jumper's knee and occurs in basketball players as well as field event participants in track. These knee conditions are secondary to overuse along with anatomical and functional variations from the norm. They are to be distinguished from those injuries secondary to a sudden force such as occur in the collision sports. The clipping injury in football with acute miniscal damage is well known.[19] The slowly progressive increase of pain beneath the kneecap or under the patellar tendon in a long-distance runner, is less well appreciated or understood, yet can cause considerable pain and disability.

Four conditions related to patellar malfunction have been described. Dr. Stan James, orthopedist from Eugene, Oregon, suggests that these four conditions are (1) patellar tendonitis, (2) compression syndrome of the patella, (3) subluxations of the patella, and (4) chondromalacia of the patellar. These four conditions result from varying degrees of patellar instability.

Patellar stability is dependent upon both dynamic and status stabilization. The dynamic stabilizers of the patella are the quadricep muscles, in particular, the vastus medialis, as well as the pes anserinus. The pes anserinus is the *goose-foot* arrangement of the tendinous expansions of the sartorius, gracilus, and semitendinosis muscles at the medial border of the tuberosity of the tibia. These dynamic stabilizers help prevent lateral subluxation of the patella. The static stabilizers include the following: (1) the patellar-femoral ligament, (2) the femoral condylar grooves, (3) the knee joint capsule and (4) the patellar tibial band (Figure 1).

In addition to these, there are some sexual differences and we note that a female with a wider pelvis will have a greater angle between the mechanical and anatomical axis and thus a greater frequency of patellar problems during running. A discussion of the four related patellar conditions follows.

FIGURE 1
Medical Aspect of Knee

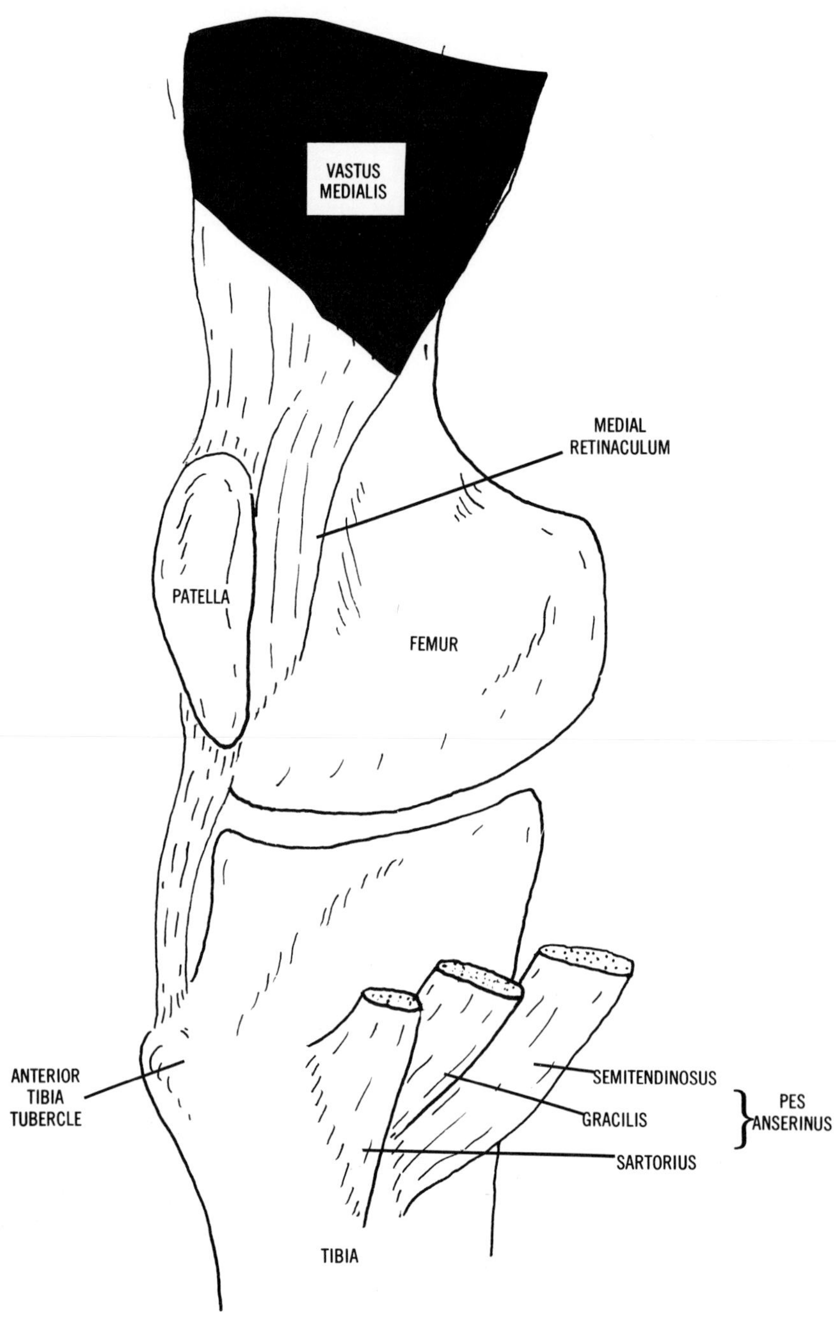

Adapted from Netter,
CIBA Series, Plate IV

PATELLAR TENDONITIS AND JUMPER'S KNEE

Patellar tendonitis occurs at the insertion of the patellar tendon and is well localized. Its etiology is secondary to traction, which is aggravated by excessive tibial torsions. Tibial torsion occurs with abnormal transverse plane rotations of the leg during compensatory foot movements in closed kinetic chain circumstances. Thus, we find an excessive internal rotation of the leg with closed kinetic chain pronation, and external rotation of the leg during compensation for an internal hip position or metatarsus adductus. Torsion affects the angle between the inferior patellar pole and the anterior tibial tubercle which aggravates the patellar tendon at its insertion (Figure 2 A & B).[2]

FIGURE 2A
JUMPERS KNEE

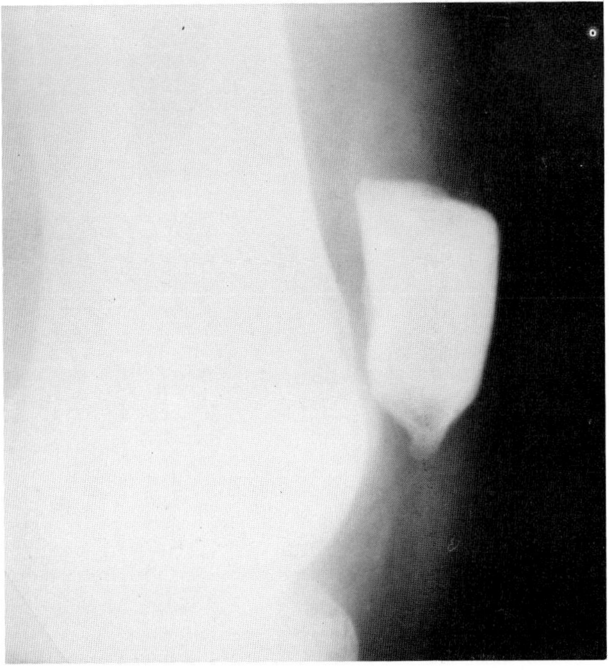

FIGURE 2B
CHONDROMALACIA OF KNEE

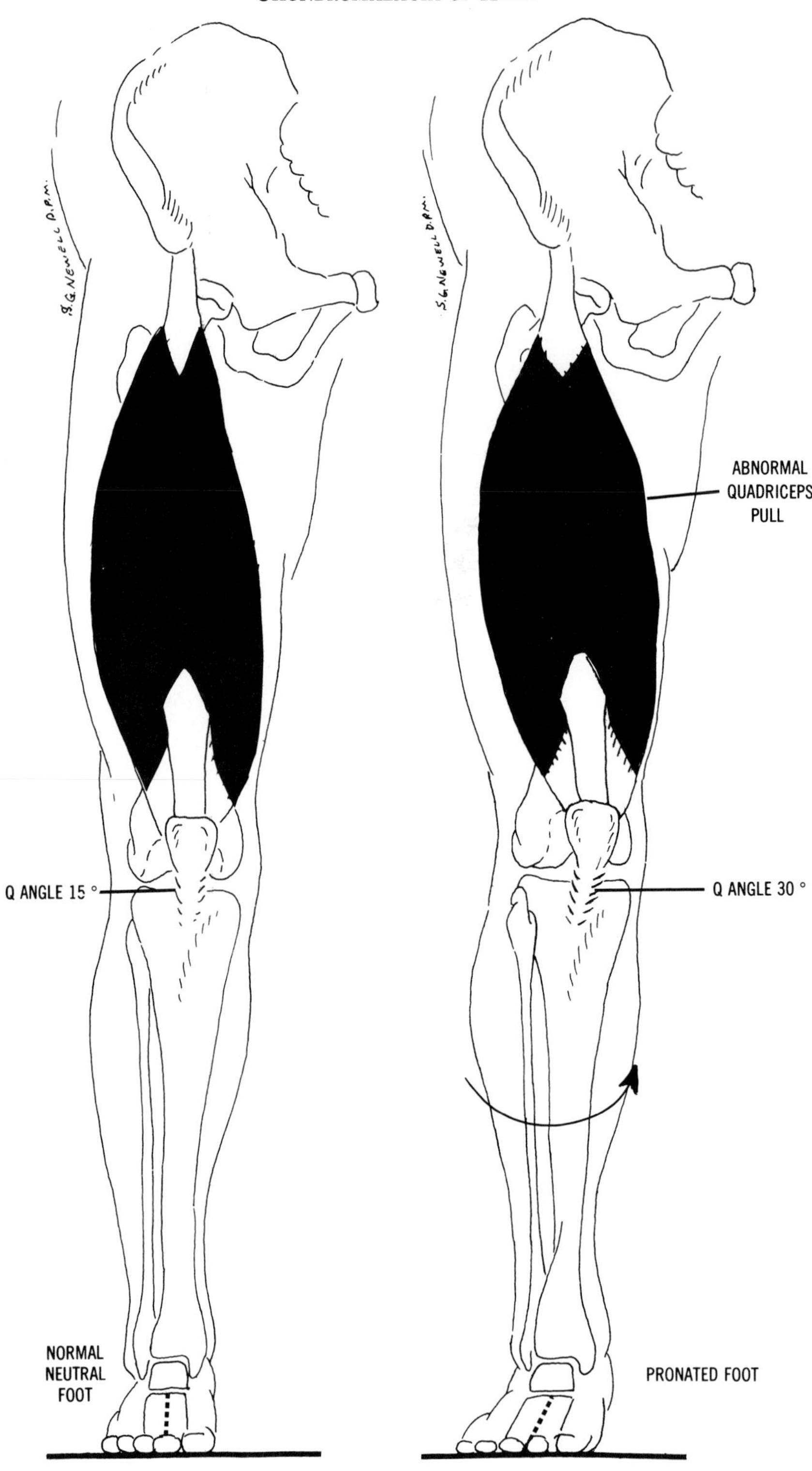

Jumper's Knee, as described by Blazina et al.,[2] may occur at the superior or inferior patellar pole regions. The athlete is almost always involved in some type of repetitive activity, such as jumping, climbing, kicking, or running. During these activities, it is assumed that the athlete is placing at least enough stress on the knee extensor mechanism to cause microtearing of the attachments of the tendon to the bone. This microtearing may occur in basketball, volleyball, high-jumping, long-jumping, triple-jumping, platform diving, cross country running, mountain climbing, football (place kicking), figure skating or tennis. An aching type of pain usually disappears after a period of rest varying from a few hours to several days. There is a feeling of wholeness in the area of the lower tip or superior tip of the knee cap. A sensation of weakness may be noted, but this is momentary and does not approach a true locking or catching. On rare occasions, the onset may be related to a discrete injury during a take-off (or landing) followed by the development of persistent aching in the knee. In the younger athlete, one may obtain a history of recent rapid growth.

Symptoms initially are aching which appears at the beginning of an activity, and disappears after warming up. Pain may then reappear after competition or activity. With progression of injury, the aching becomes more persistent and remains present before, during, and after activity. In the final stages, there is definite impairment of performance and the athlete becomes quite apprehensive about further participation in sports. From this final stage, it is possible to go a complete rupture of the patellar tendon.[2]

Specific signs include exquisite tenderness upon palpation of the inferior or superior pole of the patella. Other patellar signs, such as laxity and chondromalacia, may be present. Generally, there are no findings which suggest a meniscal or ligamentous derangement.[21] Distance runners with this problem, traditionally, have weak quadriceps which may be associated with abnormal pronation of the lower extremity during running. There may have been a history of Osgood-Schlatter Disease or patellar chondromalacia. Genu recurvatum or genu valgum may be present. Abnormal transverse plane rotations of the leg are a constant finding.

Blazina has pointed out that x-ray examination should include anterior-posterior, lateral, intercondylar, and patellar tangential (Hughston) views. Initially, the films may be negative, or one may note only a radiolucency at the involved pole. Eventually, calcification at the insertion of the tendon or a stress fracture may be present (Figure 2A).[2] Treatment consists of rehabilitative exercises including combinations of isometric and isotonic exercises for strengthening the extensors of the knee.[16] In addition, abnormal pronation should be controlled with a functional foot device.[37] For mild to moderate problems, which have pain either before or somewhat after running, but no problem during running, we utilize ice massage twice a day, along with the above modalities. When there is pain during and after an activity, rest is suggested along with exercises until such a point that activity may be resumed without pain.

Results for this problem, utilizing functional foot control, proper conditioning and training procedures, icing, and elastic wraps during the initial stages, have been relatively good. It has been unnecessary to use anti-inflammatory oral medications for these problems and only rarely have cortico-steroid injections been used. Local injections of steroids are certainly not recommended for any acute conditions.

For those more severe problems which do not respond well to conservative treatment, referral to orthopedic surgeons is called for and they have reported that decompression of the patellar tendon, as well as occasionally excising calcified tendons, gives good results. Generally, the orthopedists feel that excision of portions of the patella have less favorable results. I have had some patients with jumper's knee and extreme laxity of the patella, who are resistant to conservative treatment. My female patients with weak extensor mechanisms of the knee appear to be treated less successfully for this problem by conservative measures. Their incurred coxa vara is postulated as a factor.

PATELLAR COMPRESSION SYNDROME

Patellar compression syndrome is very similar to chondromalacia of the knee except the cartilage of the patella is normal.[14] There is usually a tightness of the vastus lateralus. The lateral retinaculum of the knee is also tight. Symptoms are similar to that of chondromalacia, but there is less discomfort. Treatment consists of functional control of the foot, as well as quadricep exercises to build up, in particular, the vastus medialis. When conservative treatment fails, Dr. James has reported that a lateral retinacular release gives good results. Other stabilizing surgical procedures may be necessary.[28]

SUBLUXATIONS OF THE PATELLA

When lateral subluxations of the patella occur, there are symptoms similar to meniscus problems. The patients complain of catching, swelling, grading, and stiffness about the knee cap.[20] As these problems progress, there is pain during and after running. The pain may be so severe that it interferes with normal walking. There is stiffness when sitting and standing and also during driving. Swelling about the patella may be present.

Physical examination often reveals abnormal function of the foot as well as deviations of the leg itself, including genu recurvatum. There is lateral displacement of the patella with sitting secondary to either an anatomical or functional problem. The patella may rest in a shallow femoral groove, which predisposes to lateral subluxation. An excessive "q" angle is formed between the inferior patellar pole and the anterior tibial tubercle (Figure 2B). Tangential patellar views will show lateral subluxation of the patella. The fulcus angle, between the patella and femoral condyles is increased.

Treatment consists of isometric quadricep exercises as well as elastic knee braces with lateral felt buttress to prevent lateral subluxation. It may be necessary to utilize a cylinder cast from four to six weeks. Following this, the athlete should resume activity while wearing functional foot supports and a long elastic knee support. A felt horseshoe pad, may be utilized with this elastic support. The runner is advised to stay on flat surfaces and avoid hills. Exercising with flexed knee positions is ill-advised. Eventually, shortened distances are stretched into longer distances and the runner can change his activity from level surfaces to gently, rolling surfaces. It is important to use shoes with thick heels that have good shock absorbing properties. This common sense approach to training and conditioning, as well as controlling the abnormal function with orthotics, has given very good results for this problem.

In those patients who are totally refractory to conservative treatment, orthopedic surgeons suggest either cessation of the athletic activity or surgical procedures including lateral retinacular releases and anterior tibial tubercle transfers.[14, 28]

CHONDROMALACIA OF THE PATELLA

Chondromalacia of the knee (runner's knee)[24] is an extremely common condition secondary to jogging and running. It is present as a grating sensation with fullness and pain beneath the knee cap. This may be present in the morning and more prevalent after sitting for prolonged periods of time. There is pain walking up and down stairs. First, the pain is exercise related. It progresses to pain during walking as well as running activities. Pain may even be present while pushing the clutch during driving.

Physical examination reveals a positive squeeze test when the patient is asked to contract the quadriceps mechanism with the knee extended. Pressure over the kneecap during this contracture elicits extreme pain. Lateral mobility of the patella is noticed. An obliquity between the inferior pole of the patella and anterior tibial tubercle is noted (Figure 2). These athletes, traditionally; have relative weakness of the anterior muscles of the thigh. Abnormal pronation of the foot, with secondary abnormal transverse plane rotations of the leg, is a common finding. Findings consistent with meniscal damage or ligamentous injury to the knee, are absent.[20]

X rays may show a patellar *baja,* with a low-riding patella. Tangential (Hughston) views may show lateral patellar tilting or displacement.

Chondromalacia of the knee is a gradual wearing down of the cartilage on the under surface of the patella. Although some wearing of the cartilage occurs normally from the age of twenty it is accentuated in the athlete with chondromalacia. There may be fracturing and fissuring of the cartilage which leads to scarring and irregularities of the various joint surfaces.

Treatment consists of establishing functional neutral control of the foot, as well as sound training and conditioning principles. Isometric as well as isotonic quadricep exercises are vigorously carried out. "Quad sets" are done with toes pointing in, and wearing a knee brace in advanced cases. Isometric quadriceps contractions (quad sets) are held for the count of twenty, twenty at a time, carried out at least twice a day. Isokinetic machines are beneficial. In addition, straight leg raises are carried out forty times a day with feet adjusted utilizing graduated weights on the feet up to ten pounds. No bent knee weight training or exercising is allowed. In most instances, chondromalacia of the knee has responded quite well to this treatment program. In cases that do not respond to this therapy, orthopedic surgery is indicated. Race walking appears to have no knee injuries and may be a sensible alternative.

SUMMARY

In summary, I have described four related patellar conditions secondary to athletic involvement and overuse syndromes. By and large, these problems are best treated by combinations of proper training, conditioning, and biomechanical control of the lower extremity. When these patellar conditions do not respond to this approach, it is proper to have consultation with a sports-minded orthopedic surgeon for further treatment.

Chapter 15

Soft Tissue Disorders of the Foot and Leg

INTRODUCTION

Soft tissue disorders of the foot and leg include strains, sprains, tendonitis, combinations of bursitis, myositis, fasciitis, and periostitis, as well as various nerve entrapments and compression. Also included under the soft tissue problems are those of verrucae. The cutaneus disorders, secondary to abnormal pressure points and shearing forces will be considered under the topics of bony disorders which are the etiological factors in the various corns, callouses, and keratomas of the foot.

STRAINS

A strain is a tear in the muscle-tendon complex. Strains are generally graded first degree if they are mild to minimal, second degree if moderate, and third degree if there is a complete disruption in the muscle-tendon unit. Unless there is a complete rupture of the myotendinous unit, there is really no accurate way to tell how severe a strain is. The amount of pain, swelling and spasm help make the classification as to first or second degree deformity.[6]

First degree injuries tend to heal more readily and allow for early return to full training than do second degree injuries. A second degree injury must be treated cautiously, inasmuch as it may progress to a third degree strain. In addition, a second degree strain, if allowed to go untreated, may result in excessive scar formation with delayed healing.[29]

Rifts of the myotendinous units heal by fibrosis of these inelastic type tissues and are in need of constant flexibility and stretching exercises before participation in sports. Failure to do so may be inviting further injury as well as constant pain during running.

One of the more common strains occurring with runners is that of the myotendinous junction of the tendo Achillis. There may also be partial ruptures of the gastrocnemius or soleus muscle bellies. These are usually palpable as actual defects or rifts in the muscle-tendon units. There is severe pain with direct and side-to-side pressure. It is best to examine the muscle-tendon units with the patient doing an isometric contraction against the examiner's body while the examiner palpates the muscle-tendon masses.

A more chronic type of strain occurs with a myositis and periostitis combination in the anterior or posterior compartments. These are commonly known as shin splints. Depending on the location of the actual shin splints, a tendonitis may also be involved. There is generally pain with pressure over the involved compartments and especially pain with movement of the involved tendon. The posterior tibial tendon, as well as the remainder of the flexor group appears to be involved most often in those athletes with a chronic pronatory problem. The chronic pronation especially places the posterior tibial muscle under undue stress which causes a partial rupture and/or a periostitis at the muscle attachment to the tibia. The flexor hallucis longus tendon may be involved secondary to a push-off problem during jumping and running. The anterior compartment is involved often times with shin splints which begin as the runner first starts vigorous training. The anterior tibial muscle and extensors are decelerators of the foot at heel contact. The athlete, unaccustomed to a vigorous heel contact, may overutilize these muscles at first as he attempts to decelerate the foot at impact on the running surface. We often note anterior shin splints as the runner goes from a track outdoors, to running on indoor boards. All of the shin splint problems must be differentiated from a compartment syndrome which is characterized by a progressive woody-type firm edema in a closed-spaced compartment. In the case of the compartment syndrome, the skin becomes reddened and the compartment is exquisitely tender.[31] This is a progressive problem with eventual neurological damage. The sports medicine physician should never allow the compartment syndrome to progress to such a state that neurologic damage is evident. If the compartment syndrome appears to be progressing an emergency fascia release is indicated. Nonresponsive "shin-splints" may actually be stress fractures of the tibia or fibula which respond to eight weeks of rest. X rays will show healing fractures six to twelve weeks following injury.

The treatment of the myositis, periostitis, or mild impending compartment syndromes is that of rest, elevation, and ice. In addition, the patient should be observed for any progression of the myositis or intracompartmental edema. Following the application of ice for the first 24 to 48 hours, which is done four to five times a day, the patient is gradually allowed to utilize gentle passive resistive exercises. These are often done over ice. The first degree injuries heal more readily and the athlete may return to running within one to two weeks. The second degree injuries take from three to four weeks before the athlete may return to athletic endeavors. It is important that flexibility exercises be continued as well as strenghtening exercises, prior to and after athletic endeavors.

A complete rupture will require either total immobilization in plaster of paris for four to six weeks, or an open surgical reanastomosis.

Many of the strains of the lower extremity are secondary to improper functioning of the foot and it is always advisable to find a biomechanical explanation for the injury and correct the etiology with a functional orthotic. When initially returning to running or competition it may be advisable to use protective strappings and various felt paddings, depending on the sport. For running sports, it is always advisable to use a functional type orthotic, or a soft orthotic if faster speeds are being employed.

SPRAINS

Sprains are basically a tear in a ligament. Ligaments occur around joints and have as their primary function that of limiting excessive normal ranges of motion. Ligaments do not function well to limit abnormal motions occurring around a joint. Ligamental sprains can be classified as first, second, or third degree sprains. Not all third degree sprains need surgery, but they all need some form of complete immobilization.[6]

In runners, the most common sprain is the first or second degree sprain of the lateral collateral ligaments of the ankle. Most common is the anterior collateral ligament. First degree sprains consist of a partial or complete disruption of the anterior collateral ligament of the ankle joint on the tibular side, and should be treated with ice and elevation for 24 to 48 hours, followed by three to four days of rest.

The second degree sprain will have pain over two of the lateral collateral ligaments and the resting period is up to six weeks, depending on the number of ligaments torn. The second degree sprain should be treated, initially, with ice and elevation. Because of the amount of swelling present, it may be necessary to utilize nonweight-bearing with crutches and ace wraps until the swelling decreases. A good guide as to when training can resume is the amount of pain with digital pressure over the lateral collateral ligaments. If there is any pain to pressure, no jogging or running should be allowed.

Third degree sprain of the lateral collateral apparatus involves complete disruption of the whole apparatus and there is a positive drawer sign. This is determined when the examiner stabilizes the anterior surface of the leg and then displaces the whole foot, anteriorly. When this maneuver is possible, then the posterior lateral collateral ligament is disrupted. Third degree sprains require immobilization for three to four weeks in either a posterior splint or below-the-knee well padded walking cast. Following this, physical therapy should be employed and gradual resumption of athletic endeavors can be gauged by the absence of pain over the lateral collateral ligaments. Some authorities prefer to do an open surgical repair of the ligaments when a third degree sprain is present.

TENDONITIS

Tendonitis is basically an inflammation of the tendon. There may also be an inflammation of the tendon sheath. Probably the most common tendonitis seen in sports medicine is that of the tendo Achillis. Other common areas of injury are the posterior tibial tendon as well as the peroneal tendons. The anterior tibial tendonitis is commonly seen with a shin splint type problem. This tendonitis can be secondary to a direct blow to the tendon with secondary inflammation of the tendon sheath or it may be secondary to partial tears in the tendon which cause a secondarily inflammatory process to occur to enable the tendon to heal. Mature tendons have no active fibroblast of their own and they require migration of healing elements from outside the tendons. This causes an inflammatory process in the tendon sheath, itself, which narrows the orifice in which the tendon glides. If the tendon is not properly rested, a vicious cycle is set up whereby a tendon moving in the inflamed sheath caused increased tendonitis.

Initial treatment for tendonitis requires ice applied four to five times a day for approximately 25 minutes for the first 24 to 48 hours. Rest and elevation and ice will all act to diminish the swelling. Local cortico-steroids should not be utilized in this initial phase inasmuch as they will retard the healing of the injured tendon. As a general rule, the greater the amount of swelling, the longer one can anticipate healing time will take. Following the first 48-hour ice and rest period, utilize gentle passive-resistive-stretching exercises over ice. The patient often times uses a styrofoam cup filled with ice and massages the injured part as he moves the foot through a range of motion placing the tendon on a moderate amount of stretch. When tenderness has subsided, begin with more vigorous passive-resistive-stretching exercises to build up flexibility and strength. This is only carried out after there is no pain with this type of motion. It will then be very important for the athlete to do proper flexibility exercises prior to any athletic endeavor. Failure to do so will invite a recurrence of the tendonitis. Once a tendon problem has occurred, there is an increased chance for its recurrence in the athlete. The athlete must find a shoe with a proper heel which appears to not aggravate the tendonitis, especially in the case of the tendo Achillis problem. Any sudden change from a higher heeled shoe to a lower heel competitive shoe could lead to a recurrence. Initially, the tendo Achillis tendonitis should be treated with a neutral functional orthotic as well as a heel lift. This heel lift is gradually reduced as stretching and flexibility exercises are increased. The posterior tibial tendonitis occurs secondary to chronic pronation and should be treated with a functional orthotic to control the chronic pronation. For some sports, it may be necessary to utilize various forms of strapping, with medial arch pads to prevent this abnormal pronation. The anterior tibial tendonitis responds well to exercises to build up the anterior tibial muscle following the episode of tendonitis. Initial treatment might include sponge under the ball of the foot to decrease the shock of foot contact and thereby lessen the need for the anterior muscle group to undergo violent contractions. In addition, it appears as though the anterior muscle group is involved in overuse problems when there is excess of forefoot pronation taking place. It may be that the anterior group tries to prevent this pronation by acting as a supinator about the midtarsal joint longitudinal axis. In these instances, biomechanical foot controls are indicated.

There have been cases of peroneal tendonitis, secondary to an actual lateral foot compression syndrome. In these cases, the pronation of the foot, through the lateral counter of the shoe, aggravates the peroneal tendon. The peroneal tendons can furthermore be actually compressed by the bone elements of the lateral aspect of the heel during abnormal pronation. Treatment consists of functional orthotics.

When a flexor hallucis longus tendonitis is present, it responds well to strappings of the great toe to disallow excessive extension. Follow-up treatment is with various forms of crest pads to enable the toes to have more of a gripping effect.

Tendonitis occurring around the medial and lateral hamstrings is common in patients who fail to do proper stretching exercises. In runners, the hamstrings, as well as all posterior muscles, become very tight and there is a constant need for flexibility exercises to prevent the tendonitis which occurs from excessive overutilization of the posterior muscle groups. Following an initial icing period, gradual flexibility exercises should be instituted and this generally takes care of the hamstring problems, providing they are not too severe.

There are those tendon problems which never receive proper primary treatment and linger on to become chronic problems. In these cases, healing has already been taking place in regard to the rift within the tendon. The problem is the chronic inflammation of the tendon sheath. In these cases, the judicious use of local long- and short-acting cortico-steroid mixtures may be indicated. In addition, proper flexibility exercises should be carried out as well as biomechanical treatment of any foot abnormality. Those tendon problems not responding to this form of therapy may need surgical intervention. Surgical decompressions of very tight tendon sheaths are generally benign procedures and have rather good results. The athlete may return to competition within four to six weeks following one of these procedures.

Among tennis players, it is not uncommon to have a ruptured or strained plantaris tendon. This is rather an unimportant tendon and no treatment other than rest is really necessary. Although this is a painful problem, the pain should resolve itself within three weeks. Relief of pain will be aided by the use of heel lifts and strappings of the foot in an equinus position. The initial symptoms of this problem include a rather sharp pain at the medial aspect of the posterior superficial muscles of the leg. It is sometimes difficult to distinguish the ruptured plantaris from a second degree problem of the soleus muscle or medial head of the gastrocnemius muscle. All of these injuries of the posterior group do respond well to icing for the first 48 hours and then resting with the foot in an equinus type position.

Returning to Training Following Tendon Injuries

FIRST DEGREE INJURIES

It was stated previously that tendon injuries can be classified as first, second or third degree. A first degree tendon injury is basically a tendonitis and may be caused by a sudden change in routine, such as from flats to spikes. A changing in the surface from grass to cinder or in training from endurance to speed, may cause a tendonitis. In addition, we have noted that a tendonitis may be secondary to biomechanical problems in the foot which place undue stress on various tendon units.

The symptoms of tendonitis are those of pain and stiffness an hour or so following activity, particularly after rest. There may be swelling which is initially difficult to detect. The examining physician will find pain with contraction and stretching of the muscle-tendon unit as well as tenderness to squeezing over the particular tendonitis area. Walking is possible, running difficult, and sprinting impossible. Return to activity may be allowed when the activity causes no pain. A basic rule of thumb is that if there is a little bit of stiffness and pain prior to activity which goes away during the activity, and then may return again after the activity, very little damage has been done by the activity and as long as proper stretching exercises and icing are carried out, the tendonitis should recede on its own.

SECOND DEGREE INJURIES

Second degree problems include partial ruptures, in which case the etiology may have been a sudden explosive act or the sequella of long-standing tendonitis and overuse syndrome.

The symptoms include the onset of pain during activity with obvious swelling apparent following the activity, usually within one hour. There is pain with contraction of the muscle unit which is even more severe with any stretching. There is a great deal of pain with squeezing over the actual area of partial rupture. Walking is difficult, and running other than the very slowest jog, is impossible. Partial ruptures must be allowed to heal by fibrosis before any activity can occur. Normal fibrosis takes from three to five weeks. Following this the etiological factors must be controlled. I prefer to utilize ice massage and nonweight-bearing stretching type activities during the convalescent period. Following the convalescent period, weight-bearing stretching exercises are indicated.

THIRD DEGREE INJURIES

A third degree tendon injury is in effect a complete rupture. This can be secondary to direct blow on a tendon or can be the sequella following a second degree rupture treated improperly. In these cases, there will be muscle tendon units involved. When this occurs, initial treatment is ice and elevation for 24 to 48 hours followed by complete immobilization for four to six weeks. Following this, the runner returns to activity when there is no pain involved with the activity. There must also be biomechanical evaluations in regard to functional orthotics as well as a good program of flexibility and strength exercises prior to and following all athletic endeavors.

FACIITIS

Plantar fasciitis is a common occurrence in the athlete and usually presents as pain in the plantar aspect of the foot over one of the three strips of the plantar aponeurosis. When the medial plantar aponeurosis is involved, pain is accentuated with hyperextension of the great toe. When one uses a stroking action over the medial plantar fascia, pain is accentuated. The middle strip of the plantar fascia may also be involved. It is rather uncommon for the lateral aspect of the plantar fascia to be involved (Figure 1). The plantar fascia problem may be aggravated by a coexistent heel spur and/or adventitious bursitis. In this case, the heel spur syndrome is present. The plantar fascial problems appear to be aggravated by chronic excessive pronation which places the plantar fascia on a stress or strain. Obesity also enters into the picture. Plantar fascial problems may be secondary to chronic collagen diseases.

FIGURE 1
PLANTAR FASCIITIS

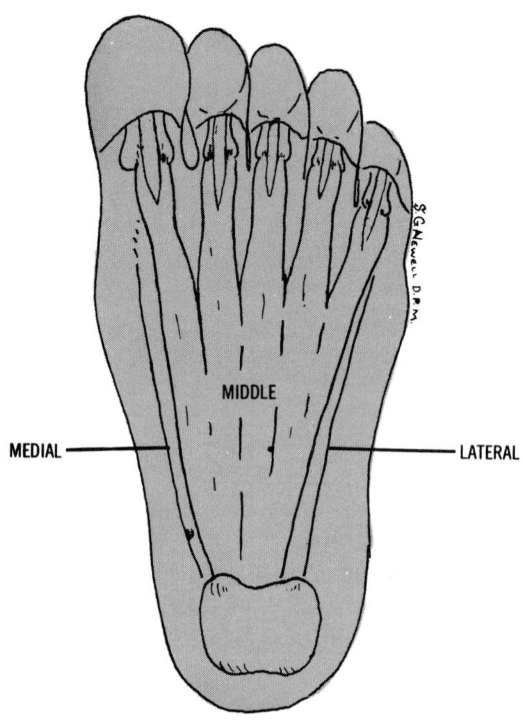

Treatment of the plantar fascial. strains and inflammatory problems consist of reversing the etiological factors by utilizing functional orthotics. When a rather severe inflammatory process is present, initial treatment should consist of physical therapy including ice massage and/or contrast baths as well as strappings of the foot to prevent excessive stretch on the plantar fascia. Chronic fascial problems may respond well to local injections of cortico-steroid preparations following which functional orthotics are utilized. X rays of the foot should be taken to verify the absence or presence of heel spur which may have to be treated in a different manner (See Chapters 16 and 17).

BURSITIS

Bursal sacs may occur over any pressure point in the lower extremity or foot. They may also occur between tendons and muscle masses or tendons and bony prominences. Bursa may be common in the upper thigh, the leg, or within the foot. Adventitious bursitis occurs in the foot most commonly over the plantar attachment of the fascia to the posterior tubercles of the calcaneus (Figure 2). This is in the area of the heel spur. This adventitious bursae is readily palpable and there is almost always pain associated with the palpation. This bursae may at times incarcerate the medial plantar calcaneal nerve and there is a combined plantar neuroma and adventitious bursae. The plantar bursae responds well to local cortico-steroid injections following which some form of foot control should be instituted. Bursae in other areas of the body, likewise respond well to intralesional cortico-steroid injections.

FIGURE 2
PLANTAR ADVENTITIOUS BURSITIS WITH NERVE ENTRAPMENT

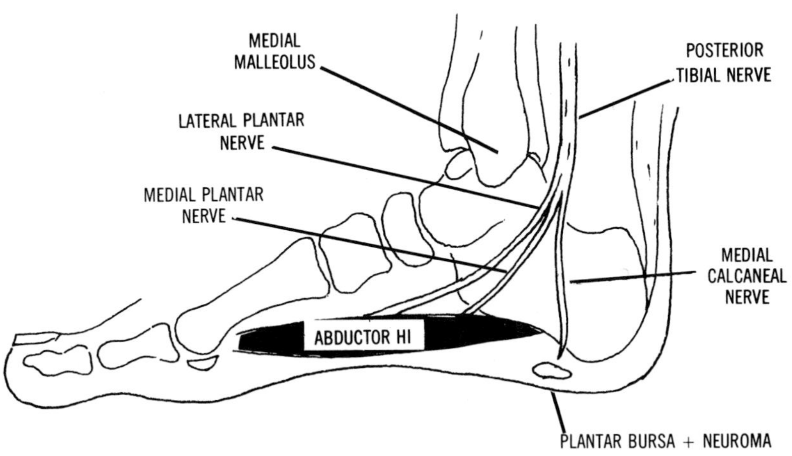

NERVE ENTRAPMENTS AND COMPRESSIONS

Interdigital Neuromas

The most common nerve problem of the lower extremity is that of the interdigital neuroma (Figure 3). The interdigital neuroma is actually an inflammation or an enlargement of the nerve sheath and it occurs most commonly in the area between the metatarsal heads and digital bases. The pain associated with the neuroma is a cramping type and is more often found in the third interspace. We have had runners with neuromas in the first, second, and fourth interspaces which were confirmed at the time of surgery, and later upon microanalysis.

FIGURE 3
Interdigital Neuroma

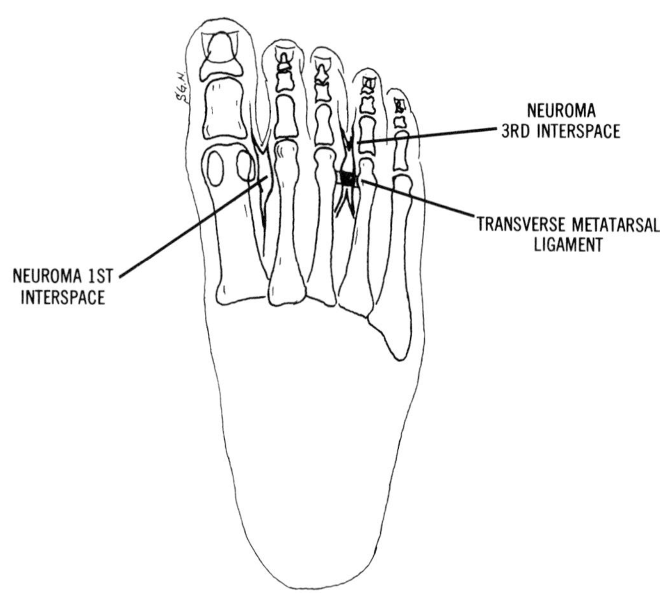

The cramping type pain must be differentiated from capsulitis and tendonitis as well as bursitis. Often there is an actual inflammatory process occurring around the nerve in which there will be an adventitious bursitis involved with the neuritis. Initial treatment consists of an injection in the interspace with a mixture of lidocaine and a cortico-steroid. In addition, biomechanical treatment is carried out to reduce abnormal metatarsal head movements which may contribute to the formation of the neuromas. Up to three separate weekly-spaced injections may be necessary. Prior to each injection, examination in the interspace area will reveal a clicking type mass which corresponds to the neuroma. Initially, there will be pain shooting both proximally and distally when this mass is palpated, but with progression of treatment, this pain should subside. The success rate with this form of conservative treatment is approximately 50%. I have had patients who have been comfortable for up to a year following this treatment and return to our office only to have the injections fail, thus necessitating eventual surgical removal of the neuromas. Surgery is rather benign and involves just local excision of the neuroma under local anesthesia.

Tarsal Tunnel Syndrome

Of the nerve entrapments and compressions seen in the athletes that have been treated, the most common is that of the tarsal tunnel syndrome. The tarsal tunnel syndrome presents a localized to radiating pain over the medial aspect of the ankle just beneath the medial malleolus (Figure 4). The tarsal tunnel is that area which, superficially, is bordered by the lacineate ligament which compresses the neuro-vascular bundles secondary to the excessive chronic pronation, inflammatory conditions of the contents of the tunnel, or localized or systemic edema problems. The floor of the tarsal tunnel is entirely bony and there is really no place for these increased space requirements to go.

FIGURE 4
TARSAL TUNNEL SYNDROME

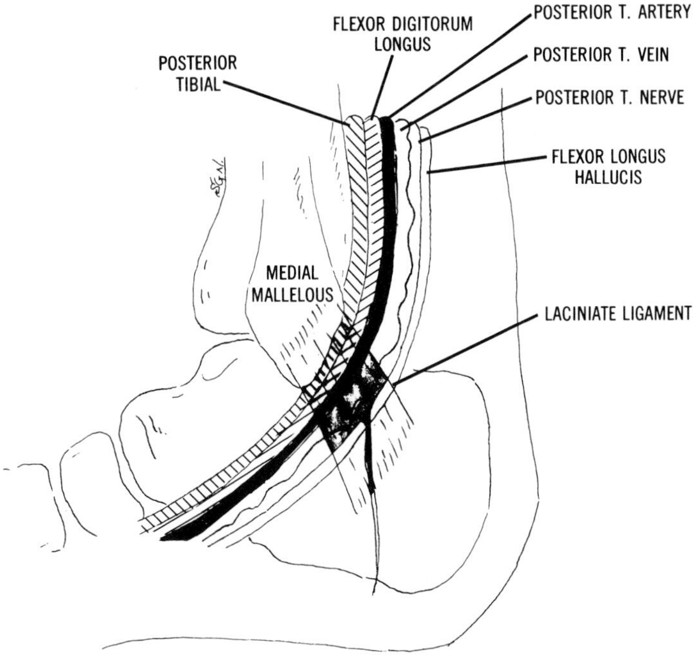

Chronic pronation causes the lacineate ligament to bow-string the tunnel with cramp-like pains occurring secondary to nerve compression. This compression may cause dilitation of the veins in the area. Advanced cases will have delayed nerve conduction studies and may demonstrate intrinsic muscular abnormalities. The pain and abnormal findings may completely be reversed following the establishment of neutral foot control. This has been demonstrated by electromyography and nerve conduction studies before and after functional foot control in patients with demonstrated tarsal tunnel syndrome.

When the tarsal tunnel is inflamed, secondary to tendonitis or phlebitis, conservative treatment appears to be less successful and a tarsal tunnel release with neuroplasty is often indicated. Thrombosed veins must be ligated during the surgical procedure. Decompression of tendons is indicated and the lacineate ligament should not be reapproximated during this procedure. The abductor canal should be freed, especially when there are medial plantar nerve entrapment syndromes.

Chronic edema, with secondary tarsal tunnel syndrome, also appears to respond less favorably to conservative treatment. Surgical decompression is often indicated.

Following surgery, a below-the-knee walking boot is applied for three weeks. If postoperative edema is anticipated, a posterior splint and nonweight-bearing with crutches is utilized.

Medial Plantar Nerve Entrapment

There may also be an isolated medial plantar nerve entrapment secondary to athletic chronic overuse. In these cases, there is pain beneath the belly of the abductor hallucis muscle or pain in the area of the long flexor tendon of the great toe. This responds to cortico-steroid injections as well as control of abnormal pronation. Should it fail to respond, a surgical neuroplasty is indicated.

Plantar Neuromas of the Heel

One of the more common nerve compression entrapment syndromes is that which occurs with the heel spur type syndrome. The heel spur type syndrome may include plantar calcaneal pain and tenderness over the heel spur area. This may be secondary to a plantar neuroma and one should suspect the medial calcaneal nerve entrapment when there is pain also at the medial aspect of the foot beneath the medial malleolus which radiates into the bottom of the foot. Physical examination will reveal tenderness over the medial calcaneal nerve which is suggestive of an entrapment syndrome. There will also be a clicking sensation of an adventitious bursae, plantarly, which appears to have the nerve entrapped within it. Histologically, this will appear as an accumulation of organized fat, bursae, and neuroma. These problems may initially respond to a medial calcaneal nerve block just distal to the tarsal tunnel area. Following this, there may be a need for local cortico-steroid infiltration into the neuroma-bursae mass. Functional foot control is always indicated to present abnormal shearing forces with abnormal pronation.

This problem must be differentiated from a plantar fasciitis or actual heel-spur syndrome.

The intractable plantar heel neuroma and/or medial plantar calcaneal nerve problem responds well to surgical excision of the neuroma with a neuroplasty of the medial cancaneal nerve.

Superficial Nerve Entrapments

Superficial nerve entrapments include those of the sural nerve and the superficial peroneal nerves. The sural nerve entrapments may follow an inversion sprain or occur with a peroneal tendonitis secondary to excessive contact pronation. This nerve entrapment is readily palpable over the course of the nerve and responds well to local cortico-steroids as well as neutral foot control. There have been times when the nerve is so extensively bound down secondary to a very bad ankle sprain or fracture that a surgical decompression has been indicated.

The superficial peroneal nerve entrapments occur most often secondary to tying the shoes too tight. There may be deep peroneal nerve pathology secondary to a tight extensor retinaculum. These generally respond well to local injections as well as padding underneath the shoe laces. When X rays reveal underlying talar neck exotosis nonresponsive cases have responded to surgery.

SUMMARY

In summation, it appears that the soft tissue injuries of the leg and foot may actually be precipitated or aggravated by athletic endeavors. The importance of proper stretching and flexibility exercises, as well as proper functional foot control is emphasized. Once a soft tissue injury has occurred, there is a likelihood that it will recur if proper preventive measures are not undertaken.

Chapter 16

Bony Abnormalities of the Foot Which Affect the Athlete

Athletes are plagued by the same bony deformities as are the more sedentary members of society. Some differences, however, are apparent. Certain activities inherent to specific sports predispose the athlete to various bony injuries or aggravate existing problems which would be less symptomatic in the nonathlete. Also, complaints which would bring a nonathlete into your office often times go unheeded by the athlete until the disability is more severe. The athlete apparently considers pain as a normal consequence of training, thus precipitating more advanced bony reactions which presumably would be checked from further progression by earlier treatment. Bony reactions to overuse, such as impingement exostosis and pressure of hyperostosis, are the end results of abnormal stresses and therefore are relatively late developments in the natural history of a deformity. It is a generally accepted principle that these later developments can be stopped by proper conservative treatment.

The excessive use of bony structures and joints is complicated by the fact that the athlete is on his feet for excessive periods of time while undergoing strenuous activity. This presents special considerations when attempting to prevent and finally correct these problems. This section will illustrate major bony deformities of the foot and will discuss those which seem to be peculiar to the athlete. Further sections will discuss the actual surgical procedures which are indicated for intractable soft tissue and bony problems.

DIGITAL DEFORMITIES

Digital deformities are either those of painful clavi over hyperostosis on relatively noncontracted toes, or pressure points and clavi over prominent bony elements of contracted toes. The soft corns overlying exostosis of the toes are generally secondary to the rubbing of adjacent toes together or the rubbing of toes against the athlete's shoe which places pressure over bony elements and results in a periostitis. This finally leads to a hyperostosis (Figure 1). These problems initially occur as an erythema of the skin, which progresses to blistering and finally callous formation. It is best for the athlete to be aware of the fact that these problems should be treated in their infancy by wide shoes with adequate room so that they do not progress to bony abnormalities. Various types of padding, utilizing felt, rubber and lamb's wool, are very useful for preventing these problems. Those digital deformities secondary to contracture are best treated by eliminating those hypermobile states of the foot which favor contracture of the toes. Imbalance of the intrinsic muscles of the toes secondary to chronic pronation should be corrected with a functional orthotic. Likewise, length pattern variations which predispose toes to trauma are best handled by utilizing neutral functional control of the foot so that a longer shoe maybe utilized without slipping of the foot within the shoe. We notice that with the so-called Morton's Foot,[35] with the long second toe, that just such a situation exists. In particular, I have noted that the varus rotated fifth toe has a particular problem in all athletes. This appears to be secondary to the fact that the shoes themselves have too much fifth toe. Along these same lines the more rigid foot gear, such as ski boots, cause particular problems over the fifth toe, as well as the fifth metatarsal heads (Figure 1). The more rigid shoe gear may predispose to digital neuromas between adjacent aspects of the fourth and fifth toes.

FIGURE 1
DIGITAL DEFORMITIES

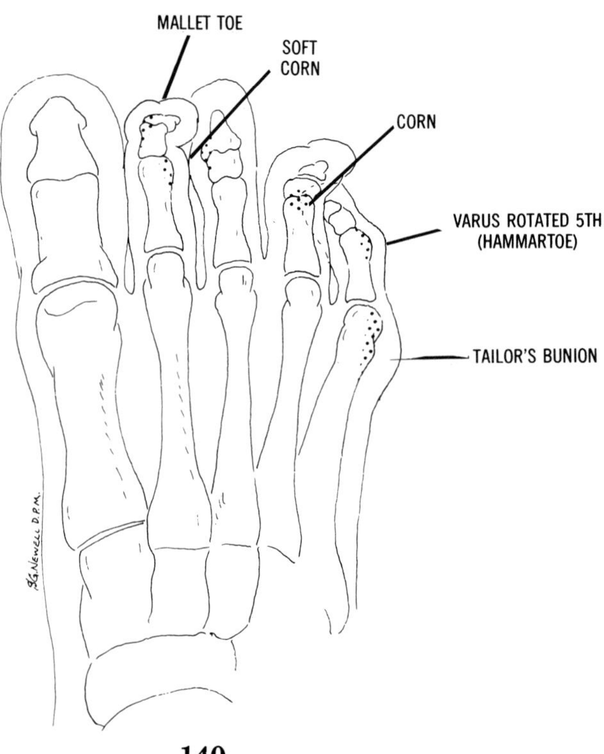

HALLUX VALGUS WITH BUNIONS

Hallux valgus with bunion deformities are secondary to hypermobility of the first metatarsal (Figure 2). In the younger athlete, erythema over the medial and dorsal aspects of the first metatarsal heads with secondarily, deviated hallux are sure signs that the hallux valgus deformity is progressing. This type of hallux valgus is often noted in the hypermobile type pronated foot with a forefoot varus. It is also more prevalent in the athlete with a very tight tendo Achillis.[32] Functional control is indicated to prevent progression in these deformities.[33] Xrays will give an indication as to the stability of the metatarsal phalangeal joints as well as the positions of the sesamoids.[10] We have had younger patients with rather severe bunions which themselves are not that painful. It is explained to these patients that instability of joint can eventually lead to arthritis which in later years will be painful. We have elected in these cases to use functional control and allow the athletes to participate in sports. When serial Xrays show progression of the hallux valgus deformity, despite neutral control, then it is advised to have a surgical realignment of the joint at a time convenient for the athlete.

FIGURE 2
HALLUX VALGUS WITH BUNION

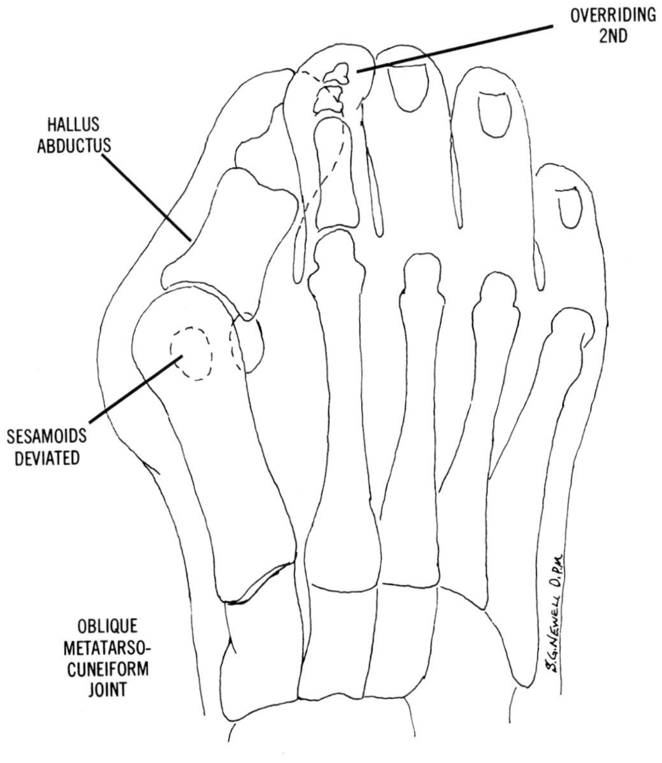

Many athletes have limitations of motion at the first metatarsal phalangeal joints with various degrees of dorsal bunions. There is no real hallux valgus present, but yet the rectus type foot predisposes to these problems. Often times the first metatarsal joint is dorsiflexed, yet not in any hypermobile state. This dorsiflexion position of a metatarsal, which is relatively plantar in regards to the adjacent metatarsals, predisposes to the dorsal bunions. Xrays reveal a dorsal hyperostosis. These problems are best treated by functional control and often a rigid forefoot valgus is the type of foot which is needed to be controlled.

TAILOR'S BUNIONS

Tailor's bunions or a hyperostosis of the fifth metatarsal head can be present with splaying of the whole fifth metatarsal or just hypertrophy of the fifth metatarsal head itself. In cases where splaying is present and the pain is significant, we advocate closing wedge osteotomies of the fifth metatarsal.[11] This will be discussed in further sections. In those cases in which only a lateral hyperostosis is present then a partial osteotomy may be carried out.[9] The Tailor's bunion causes most havoc in skiers. Ski boots are very unyielding and can actually aggravate the fifth metatarsal heads causing bursitis and hyperostosis.

PLANTAR CALLOUSES

Plantar callouses under metatarsal heads are most often secondary to shearing forces between the metatarsal heads, skin, and the shoe surface. One or two metatarsals are functioning plantar to the adjacent metatarsals. Thus, the accentuated shearing forces. These shearing keratomas are present with the hypermobile type pronated feet and the more rigid forefoot valgus feet. The keratomas are generally no problem for the younger athletes, but become more symptomatic in the middle-aged and older athletes. When we have a younger athlete who is just getting some erythema and blishering over prominent metatarsal heads, he is advised as to the problem at hand and functional control is instituted. In the patient who is a bit older with the real symptomatic intractable plantar keratomas, orthotics are advised and surgery is also indicated. The actual surgical procedures will be described in further sections.[9]

OS NAVICULARIS

I have had experiences with athletes who have a great deal of pain secondary to the os navicularis deformity. This is either a second center of ossification medial to the normal navicular or a very large projection of a styloid process of the navicular (Figure 3). This may be accentuated with a pronated foot when the posterior tibial tendon inserts in the ossicle itself somewhat dorsal to its normal attachment. It then fails to participate in the stabilization of the metatarsal joint. The athletes who complain are usually in their teens and note that they are having quite a bit of difficulty when running. The pain is secondary to pressure over the bony elements as well as posterior tibial tendonitis. Surgery is the major solution to these problems and this will be discussed in further sections.[33]

FIGURE 3
Os Navicularis and Prominent Styloid
Process of Fifth Metatarsal

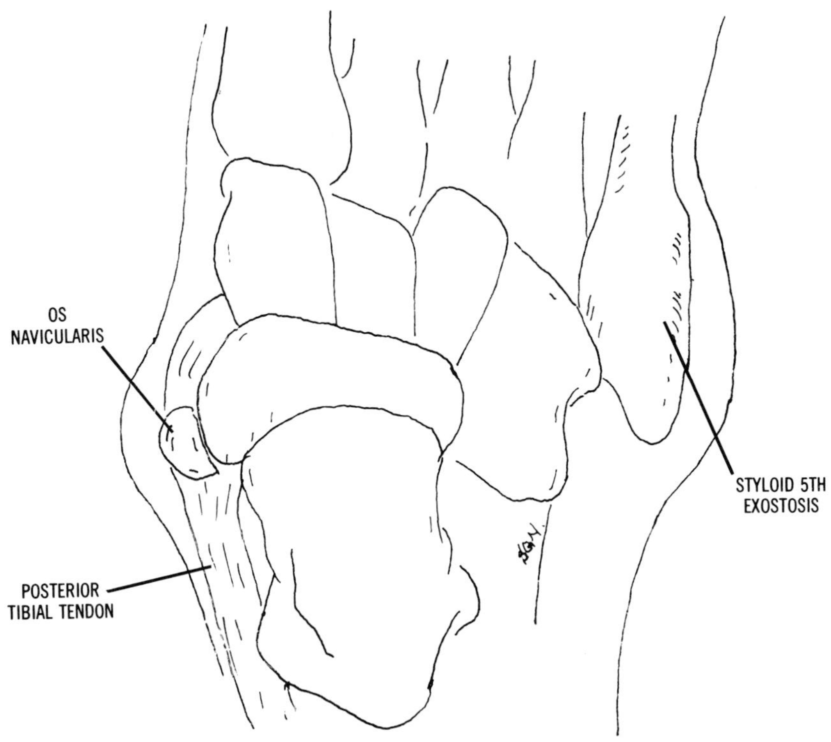

MID-FOOT EXOSTOSIS

Exostosis of the mid-foot occurs at the dorsal aspect of the first metatarsal joint secondary to impingement caused by forceful dorsiflexion of the first ray (Figure 4). These cause pain in the running gear secondary to pressure and may be associated with ganglions of the extensor tendons which cross the bony projections.[8] When padding fails to relieve the pain, surgical intervention is indicated. Likewise, the styloid process of the fifth metatarsal may become a pressure point with secondary pain associated at the attachments of the peroneus brevis tendon and the bony elements themselves (Figure 2) When these projections are quite large and associated with a forefoot or metatarsus adductus, surgical intervention often is indicated.

FIGURE 4
MEDIAL CUNEIFORM—METATARSAL EXOSTOSIS

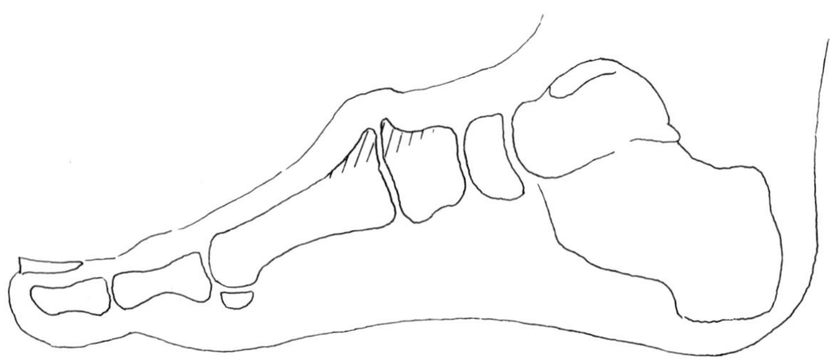

CALCANEAL SPURS AND EXOSTOSIS

Plantar Heel Spur Syndrome

The calcaneus is a frequent source of bony abnormalities in the athlete. The plantar aspect of the calcaneus is subject to a great deal of pounding trauma and stress as the foot pronates. The attachments of the intrinsic muscles of the foot at the distal aspect of the calcaneal tubercles leads to a tension reactive hyperostosis, known as the heel spur. The heel spur, in itself, may be associated with an inflammatory adventitious bursitis (Figure 5) as well as myositis, and fasciitis of those tissues surrounding it. It is best to treat these problems conservatively with neutral foot control as well as with up to three weekly-spaced cortico-steroid injections. Anti-inflammatory oral medications are generally of little value. Conservative treatment is often successful, but surgical intervention may be necessary in long-standing spurs with surrounding organized fibrosis[8] of soft tissue as well as entrapment neuromas.

FIGURE 5
HEEL SPUR

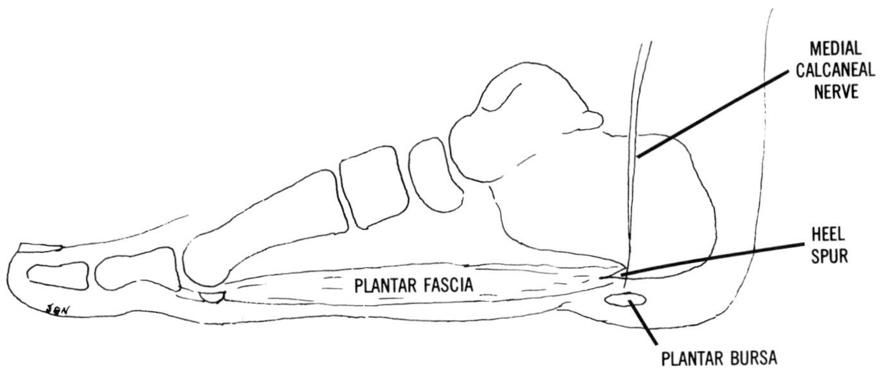

Retrocalcaneal Exostosis

The runner's bump or retrocalcaneal exostosis is a common complaint in runners.[40] The major problem is that of a stretching of the attachment of the tendo Achillis over a large projection of the calcaneus at the posterior-superior aspect (Figure 6). This retrocalcaneal exostosis is usually secondary to changes taking place at heel contact. The accentuated pronation at heel contact causes pressure over the superior-posterior aspect of the calcaneus. This eventually may lead to a reactive hyperostosis. The calcaneus, itself, may be in such a shape, intrinsically, to predispose to reactive soft tissue changes with abnormal contact stresses.

Conservative treatment consists of neutral orthotics with a rearfoot post to control heel contact. Injections of cortico-steroids may be of help and usually will not cause any soft tissue damage.

FIGURE 6
RETROCALCANEAL EXOSTOSIS (RUNNER'S BUMP)

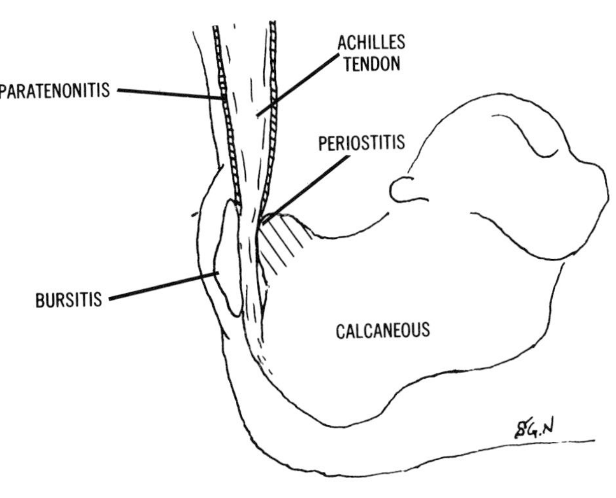

Initially, some type of padding may be useful and the back of the shoe can be cut out and elastic replaced. Despite all of this, when the problems are long standing it has been necessary to resort to surgical removal of the hyperostosis. This greatly eases the tension over the tendo Achillis and the athlete is able to participate without significant impairment of function and in a pain-free attitude. The actual surgical treatment will be discussed in further sections.

BONY DEFORMITIES OF THE TALUS

The talus is a frequently traumatized bone in sports. The talar neck often times impinges upon the anterior aspect of the tibia at the ankle joint level. This results in impingement exostosis which may have as the end result, bony limitation of dorsiflexion (Figure 7). This is sometimes referred to as jumper's ankle. You see this in long-distance runners, ice skaters, and basketball players. It has also been reported in hockey players. The talar neck exostosis, in themselves, may be symptomatic by causing abnormal pressure over neuro-vascular bundles, as well as tendons. They may predispose to entrapment syndromes and ganglion. Many times surgical intervention is the only correction for these problems.

The posterior aspect of the talus may be involved in athletic trauma secondary to abnormal pressures over the os trigonum. The os trigonum may be a free ossicle at the posterior lateral aspect of the talus or may be an enlarged posterior shelf of the talus itself, lapping over the posterior set of the subtalar joint. In any event, there may be a sudden pain secondary to a fracture of the os trigonum or a more nagging pain secondary to arthritic changes taking place at the posterior aspect of the subtalar joint.

FIGURE 7
TALAR EXOSTOSIS — IMPINGEMENT EXOSTOSIS OF THE ANKLE

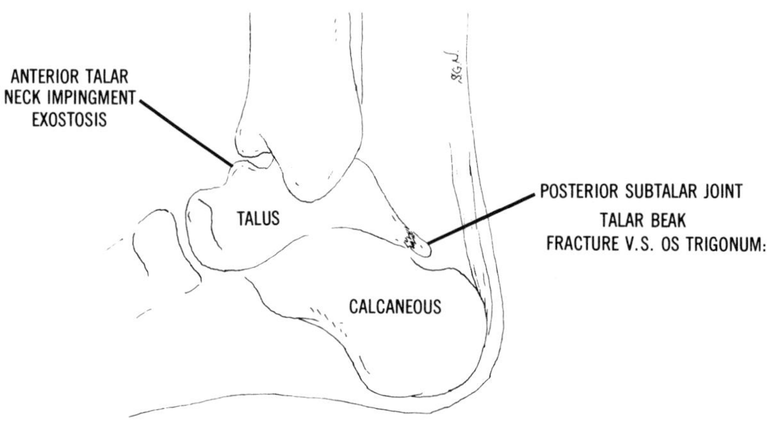

There may be changes in the range of motion of the subtalar joint when the more progressive arthritic changes are present. Radiographs are very helpful in making this diagnosis and also that of the stress fracture or extentuated posterior talus shelf. We have instances where removal of an os trigonum or resection of the posterior talar shelf has been carried out with good results. Following the surgical intervention, increased range of motion at the subtalar joint was noted and no significant impairment of function, postoperatively, was present.

SUMMARY

Presented here were those bony problems of the foot which appear to be more common in athletes. Those problems secondary to abnormal pressure over the toes, or contracture of the toe secondary to abnormal function of the foot, appear to be preventable if the athlete presents himself to the podiatrist when the deformities are in flexible states and ankylosis is not evident. Likewise, those problems of the forefoot secondary to hypermobility including intractable plantar keratomas, hallux valgus with medial bunions, and splaying of the fifth metatarsal with tailor's bunions all appear to be preventable with proper biomechancial control.

These problems of the midtarsal joint secondary to hypermobility of the forefoot, usually present themselves as exostosis dorsally at the metatarsal cuneiform level. They should be able to be prevented with functional control. Those problems at the plantar aspect of the calcaneus secondary to abnormal pronation, likewise, should respond well to early conservative treatment. The retrocalcaneal exostosis when secondary to abnormal contact pronation will also respond to conservative treatment. However, when secondary to abnormal structure of the calcaneus, itself, surgery may often times be indicated. The more advanced and long-standing the calcaneal deformity, the more likely is the failure of conservative treatment.

The impingment exostosis at the ankle joint secondary to forceful dorsiflexion of the foot at the ankle, appears to be a hazard of jumping and prolonged running. Certain foot types predispose to these problems, and in particular we note the very high arch rigid type foot. It is difficult to prevent these problems and still allow the athlete to train properly. It is likely that surgical intervention will be more frequently carried out for these problems, inasmuch as orthotics do not appear to cause major changes in the function at these levels.

Chapter 17

Surgical Correction of the Intractable Soft Tissue and Bony Abnormalities of the Athlete's Foot

INTRODUCTION

In the two preceding chapters, we have discussed those soft tissue and bony abnormalities which appear to be more prevalent among athletes. It was noted that conservative treatment for those problems secondary to abnormal foot function should result in a high success rate. It was also pointed out that the longer a deformity has been present, the greater will be the soft tissue fibrosis. In these cases conservative treatment may not be as successful. In any event, where conservative treatment fails, it is necessary to consider surgical intervention. When considering surgical intervention, the doctor must consider the advantages against the disadvantages. Will the athlete function better in sports after surgery? Is there a chance that the surgery may be either very successful and at the same time very unsuccessful? Will the athlete need to be handled in a special manner following the surgery to both protect himself from injury while allowing some form of training and exercising?

Often times surgery is the most conservative form of treatment and in as much as the athletes are in excellent condition they recover well from the stress of surgery. With the injured athlete, the surgical procedure which will give the best results, regardless of the amount of immobilization required, should be that which is chosen. An example is with the surgical corrections of metatarsus primus adductus with bunion deformity. This may be best treated via an osteotomy for the metatarsus primus adductus as well as an arthroplasty at the first metatarsal phalangeal joint for the bunion deformity.[10] In this case the athlete can well afford six weeks of immobilization in plaster to assure the best possible results.

SURGICAL PROCEDURES FOR SOFT TISSUE DAMAGE OF THE FOOT

Neuromas

Interdigital Neuromas

Neuromas more commonly occur between the third and fourth digits of the foot.[8] The neuromatous mass includes a hypertrophy of the sheath of the common plantar nerve and its two digital proper branches to adjacent aspects of the toes. This plantar nerve often times is surrounded by a hypertrophy of soft tissue with adventitious bursitis and organization of fat. (Figure 3, Chapter 15.) The neuroma may extend beneath the transmetatarsal ligament proximally, or into the bases of the toes, distally. A neuroma may occur in any interspace in the forefoot and should be considered when interdigital pain is present. Often times more than one neuroma is excised at the time of surgery.

Surgical Procedure

Neuromas are best excised with some form of hemostasis to allow for proper visualizaton of the nerve and to provide for traumatic handling of the neurovascular bundles. The nerve itself should be excised along with organized soft tissue with care being taken to preserve the venous and small arterial structures. I perfer a dorsal longitudinal skin incision for a single neuroma (Figure 1). The skin incision begins distally at the webbing of the toes and extends proximally to just behind the transmetatarsal ligament.[8] This allows for adequate exposure. This incision may be modified to allow for excision of the adjacent neuromas (Figure 1). It is somewhat futile to try to remove a neuroma through a very small dorsal incision inasmuch as an inadequate resection leads to an even more painful amputation neuroma or entrapment. Following the skin incision, utilize blunt dissection through the interspace and isolate the enlarged plantar nerve. This is freed from normal soft tissue and the proximal aspect of the nerve is traced proximal to the transmetatarsal ligament. This ligament is transected and the neuroma is resected from normal nerve. The two distal branches are then resected. The entire mass is sent to the pathologist for microanalysis. I do not utilize any deep closure in as much as normal vascular structures may be tied off. Subcutaneous tissue closure is utilized and then cutaneous closure. A compressive dressing which occludes dead space is utilized. Sutures are removed in two weeks and the athletes may begin training in three to four weeks. For the first three weeks, postoperatively, the athlete utilizes a wooden postoperative shoe which helps to splint the foot and prevents abnormal motion which might adversely affect the healing of the soft tissue.

When multiple neuromas are present, they may be excised through one or more dorsal incisions. I have used plantar incisions, transversely in an area between the metatarsal heads and bases of the toes. This is generally used on older patients. It is much preferred to stay away from plantar incisions on younger athletes.

FIGURE 1

Dorsal Incision for Adjacent Neuromas in Interspaces 2 and 3

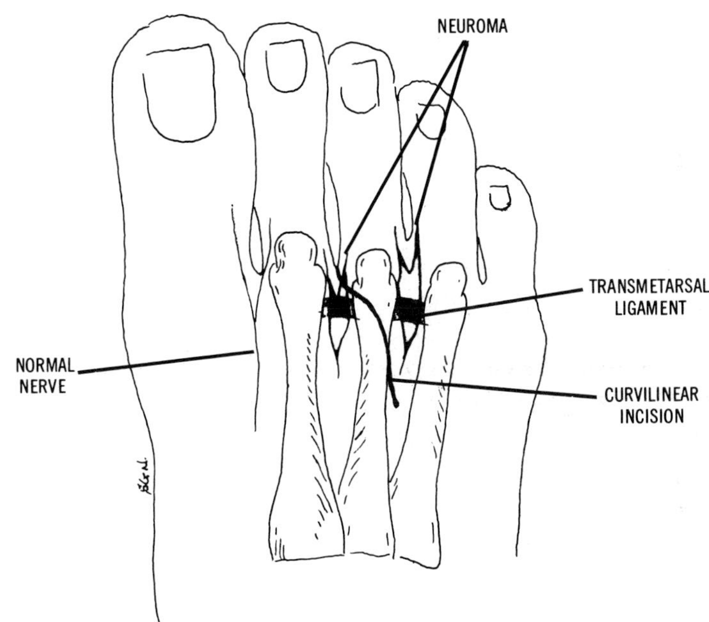

Plantar Heel Neuromas

Plantar neuromas beneath the calcaneus are secondary to abnormal compression at heel contact (Chapter 16, Figure 2). Tension may also be a factor when the medial calcaneal nerve is involved. The traction or compression neuroma is generally present at the medial plantar aspect of the foot and may be palpated as the medial plantar calcaneal nerve emerges into this soft tissue mass. It is best approached through a transverse longitudinal medial incision which is dorsal to the thick plantar skin of the foot. A dry field is necessary so that the entire soft tissue mass can be well localized by soft tissue dissection and then excised. Postoperative care is the same as for neuromas in the forefoot. It is necessary to separate this isolated problem from one involving pathology of the calcaneus itself as in the heel spur syndrome.

Nerve Entrapments

Entrapments Of Anterior Nerves Of Foot

Both the superficial and deep anterior nerves of the foot may be entrapped secondary to soft tissue constriction at the level of the extensor retinaculum or pressure from underlying bony projections (Figures 2,3,4). The superficial nerves are easily exposed through dorsal longitudinal incisions. The nerves lay in the subcutaneus fat and extensive dissection is unnecessary. It is usually possible to utilize a neuroplasty in which case the nerve is carefully separated from any restrictive soft tissue areas and moved to a healthy fatty bed. When extensive nerve damage is present, it may be necessary to sacrifice the nerve.

FIGURE 2
IMPINGEMENT EXTOSIS ANKLE

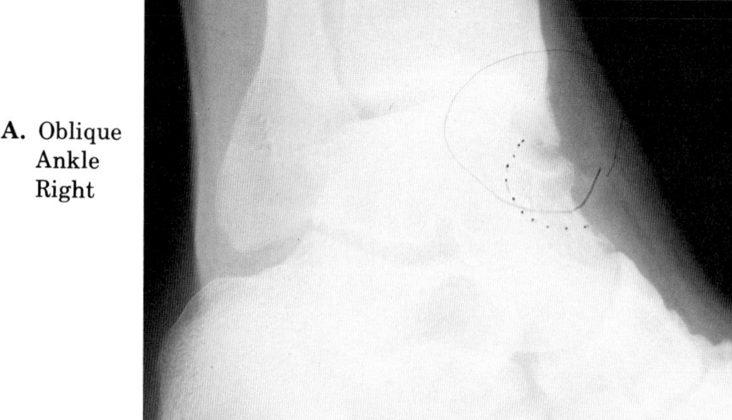

A. Oblique Ankle Right

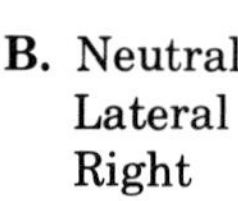

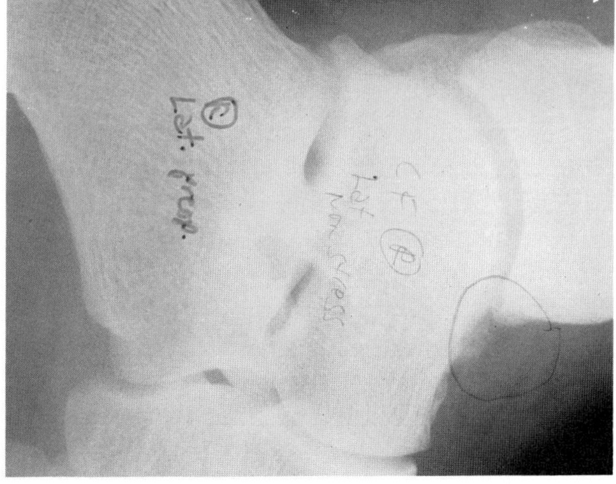

B. Neutral Lateral Right

The anterior tibial nerve is located beneath the superficial fascia and careful dissection is essential. The nerve must be separated from the anterior tibial artery and carefully freed from any soft tissue constrictive bands. Generally, a sectioning of the extensor retinaculum is sufficient to free this nerve from compression at the dorsal aspect of the foot. The extensor retinaculum is not closed in these cases. It is preferable to cast the foot for three to four weeks in a below-the-knee walking cast following this procedure to allow for maximum undisturbed soft tissue healing of the retinaculum and surrounding soft tissue structures. (Figures 2,3,4)

FIGURE 3A

Lateral Stress View, Ankle, Note Ankle Osseous Equinus

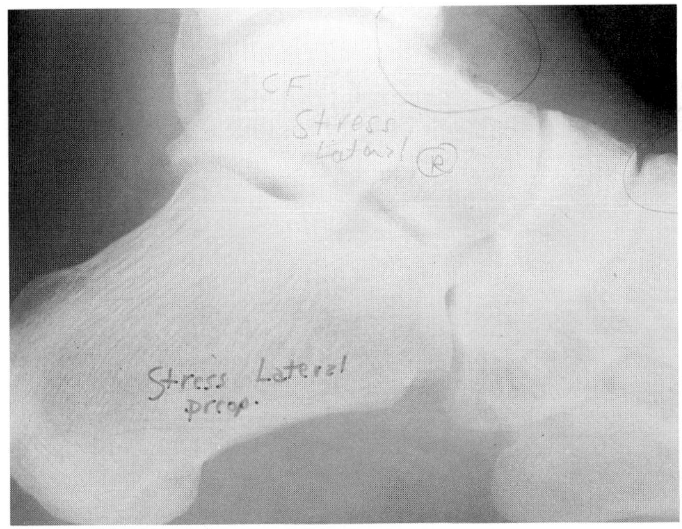

FIGURE 3B

Post Operative View right Ankle with Remodeling Talar Neck and Tibial Anterior Surface

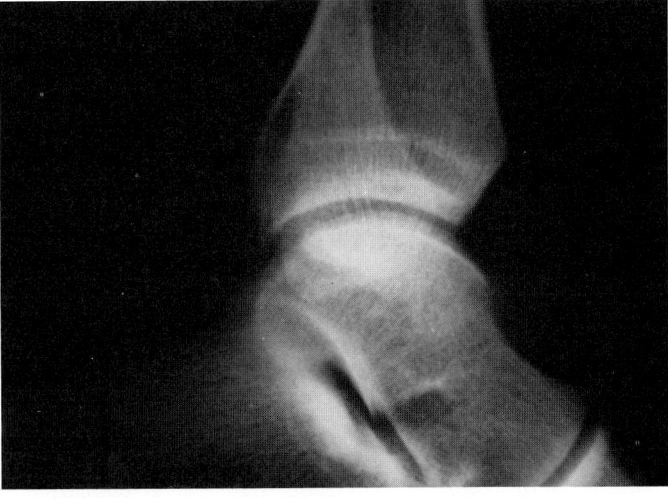

Tarsal Tunnel Syndrome

The tarsal tunnel is approached through a curved longitudinal incision which is posterior to the medial malleolus (Figure 4, Chapter 15). The neurovascular bundle is between the flexor digitorum longus and flexor hallucis longus. The flexor retinaculum must be carefully sectioned to allow for visualization of the neurovascular bundle. With the aid of blunt dissection, posterior tibial nerve and its branches at the trifercation are identified. Restrictive soft tissue bands are freed with sharp dissection. Veins in this area may be dilated. When the veins are thrombosed it is best to ligate them high. It is important to free both the proximal aspects of the tarsal tunnel, as well as the abductor canal. The medial calcaneal nerve may be involved, in which case the incision must be extended, distal medially, and the nerve localized between the abductor muscle and the long flexors. A neuroplasty is generally sufficient for freeing this nerve. There have been instances of neurmas of the medial plantar calcaneal nerve in which case resection is indicated. In the isolated tarsal tunnel syndrome, neuroplasty is sufficient and the flexor retinaculum should not be reapproximated. Closure of subcutaneous tissue and skin is all that is required. A compressive dressing should be placed and a below-the-knee walking cast is utilized from four to five weeks. Abnormal swelling may be indication for bivalving the cast in the early stages following surgery. If postoperative edema is anticipated a posterior splint is preferred for the first postoperative week.

Chronic Tendonitis

Chronic tendonitis with construction of the tendon sheath which fails to respond to conservative treatment including rest, cortico-steriod injections, and neutral foot control, are well approached by decompression surgically (Figures 5 and 6). Incisions are planned to afford maximum visualization of the tendon sheaths, which are freed by sharp dissection. These decompressions are generally met with good success. When tendon sheaths are anatomically not present, then a paratenon stripping may be carried out. This has worked especially well in cases of chronic paratenonitis of the tendo Achillis. In these cases, only hypertrophy of the paratenon has been present and the underlying tendon has been normal.

Following tendon procedures, it is generally preferable to utilize a below-the-knee walking cast for four weeks to allow for proper healing. The cast should be applied to allow reduced tension on the myotendon unit. Xerograms may aid in the diagnosis of paratenonitis or partial ruptures (Figures 5 and 6).

FIGURE 5
XEROGRAM LEFT FOOT SHOWING
OLD FRACTURE OS TRIGONUM

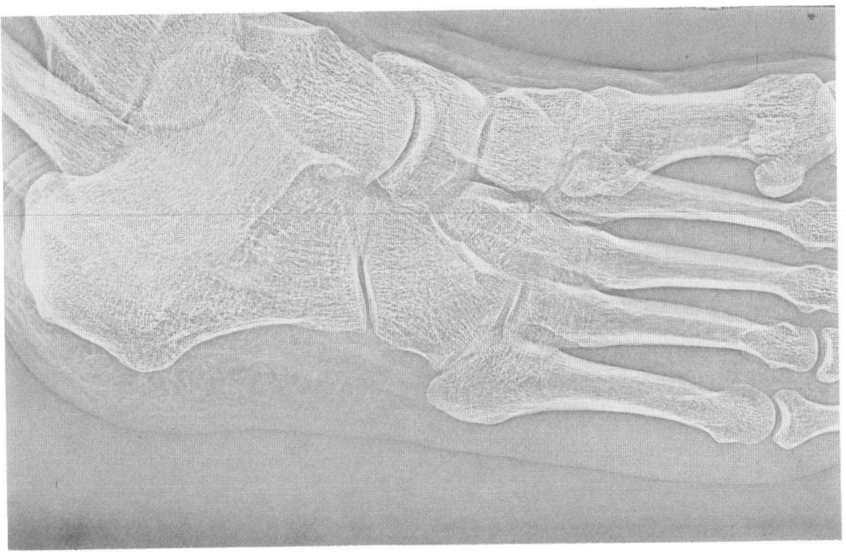

Tendo Achillis displayed a partial rupture and paratenonitis at surgery.

FIGURE 6

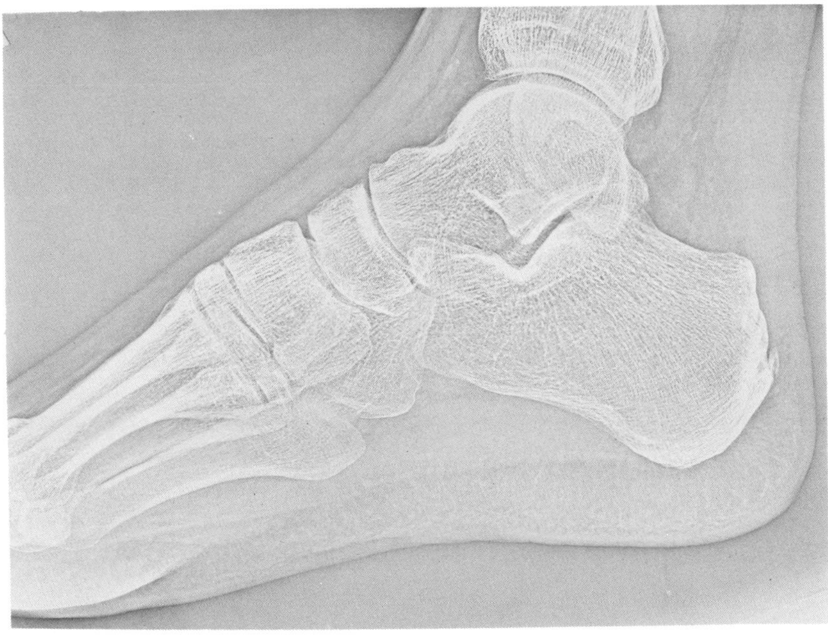

Retrocalcaneal exostosis with overlying tendo Achillis paratenonitis following severe twisting injury.

Tendon Lengthening Procedures

It has been customary to do a modification of the White[23] technique for lengthening the tendo Achillis when an anatomical shortening of the gastrocnemius is present. In these cases conservative treatment had failed despite various types of pronated and neutral orthotics. Pain was present secondary to the abnormal pronation of the foot secondary to the shortened superficial posterior muscle group. Likewise, X rays showed advanced deformity of the foot secondary to the severe pronatory forces.[32, 33] In these cases, the surgical procedure worked well, the athletes were back jogging five weeks following surgery. They progressed rapidly from the jogging stage to full activity.

Procedures For Tendo Achillis Lengthening

These cases may be done under a local anesthetic on an outpatient or inpatient basis. When outpatient surgery is performed, it is necessary to do one foot at a time, inasmuch as below-the-knee walking casts are utilized for four weeks following this procedure. A dorsal transverse skin incision is carried out just proximal to the superior aspect of the posterior surface of the calcaneus (Figure 7). This incision is placed in a skin line. With the aid of blunt and sharp dissection, the borders of the tendon are localized and defined. The anterior two thirds of the tendon are then resected with the blade somewhat obliquely angled to resect more of the fibers on the lateral aspect of the tendon. Attention is then focused on the myotendinous junction and a longitudinal skin incision is carried out at the medial aspect of the tendon. With the aid of blunt and sharp dissection, the tendon is freed, dorsally, and plantarly, with care being taken not to disrupt the tendon sheath. The medial one half of the tendon is then transected with sharp disection. With the knee extended, the foot is gently dorsiflexed and the tendon slides upon itself. It may be necessary to transect the plantaris tendon through the proximal incision if it appears to be inhibiting dorsiflexion. Both wounds are closed with a continuous subdermal suture and a below-the-knee well-padded cast is applied, with the foot being held 90 degrees to the leg. Following the removal of the cast in four weeks, the patient is allowed to gradually resume activity. While the patient is in the cast, isometric and isotonic exercises are carried out. The patient may begin training again approximately four to five weeks following surgery, but full function may not be regained for between two to three months following surgery. There is a mild amount of strength loss following this procedure which may not be totally regained for periods of up to one year. McGlamry reports good results with a recession technique to lengthen the gastrocnemius only.[17]

The decrease in pain in the posterior muscle groups and the foot itself following the tendo Achillis lengthening procedure is remarkable. One also notes radiographically that the foot begins to return to a more normal configuration. Neutral orthotics are utilized postoperatively and are tolerated in as much as the abnormal stress from the tight tendo Achillis has been released.

FIGURE 7
TENDOACHILLES LENGTHENING

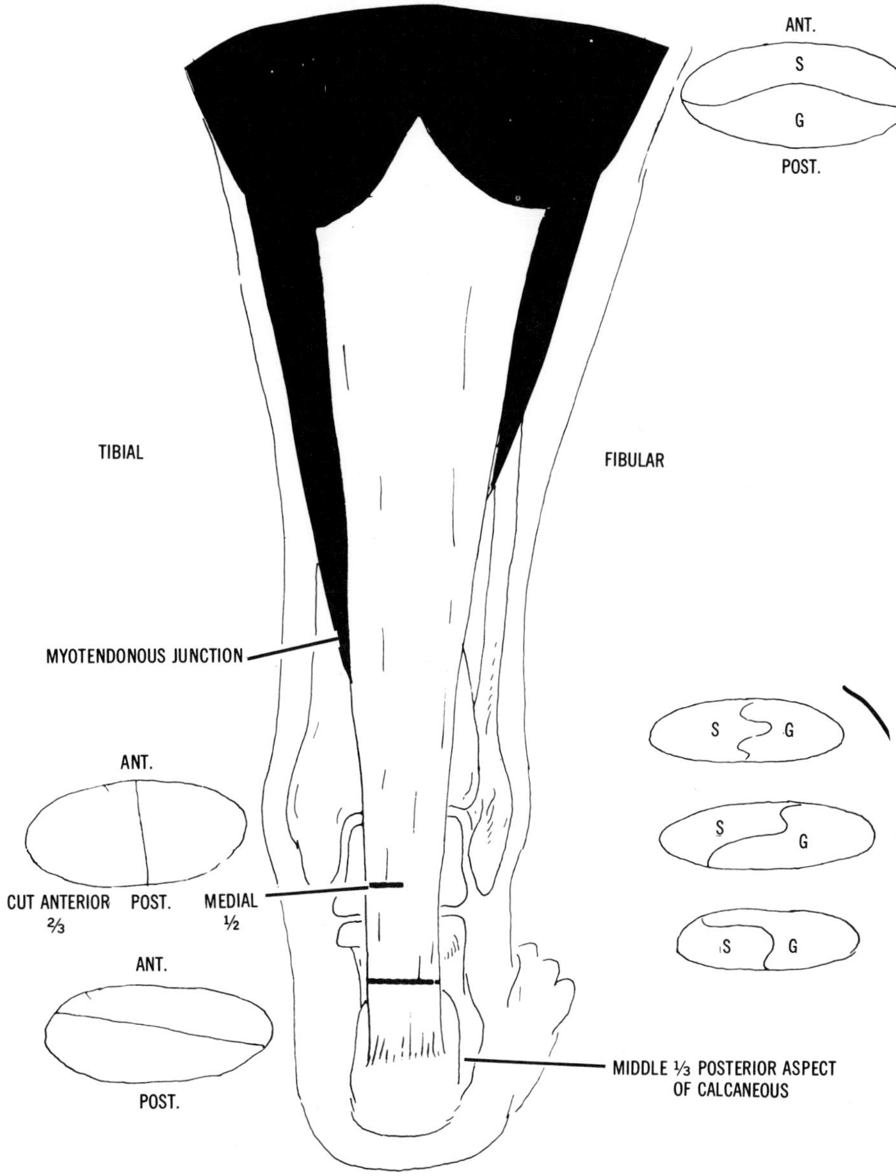

Digital Deformities

Digital deformities secondary to contracture where ankylosis is not present are often times treated well by soft tissue release of contractive tissue (Figure 8; Figure 1, Chapter 16). This usually means a flexor tendon release as well as plantar capsolotomy and an extensor release when indicated. The toes are splinted for six weeks following these procedures. The athletes are generally not able to train or run for a period of up to three weeks following surgery. The surgery is rather benign and carried out under local anesthesia in an office situation. The main reason for abstinence from activity for three weeks following surgery is to allow for proper soft tissue healing.

FIGURE 8
Digital Deformities

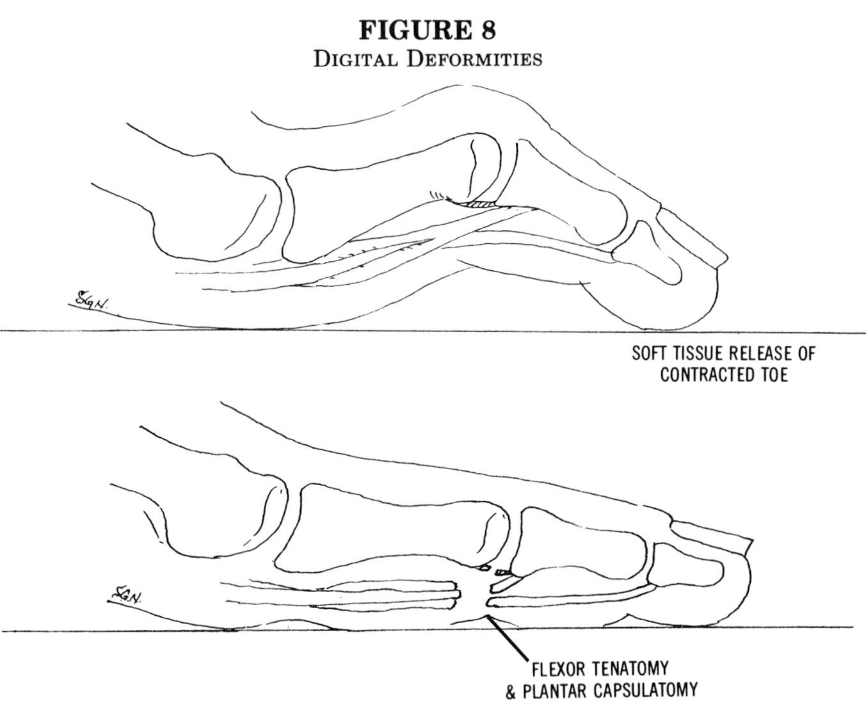

When more advanced contracture is present with evidence of joint damage it is generally preferable to utilize a resection arthoplasty with removal of the head of the proximal phalanx at the involved joint. (Figure 9). This is generally carried out through a dorsal longitudinal skin incision which is double elliptical in shape with some resection of the overlying corn. The extensor tendon is carefully handled so that it is functional following the surgery. Function may be accomplished by resuturing a section tendon or performing the arthroplasty in such a manner that the tendon is not affected. Hammer toe surgery generally keeps the athlete away from training for three weeks. Exostosis of the digits with overlying soft or hard corns are best treated by partial ostectomy. In these cases, we have used closed surgical procedures with power instruments to remove the exostosis with excellent results. These outpatients surgical procedures keep the athlete away from training for no longer than one week. We approach subungual exostosis in the same manner.

FIGURE 9
ARTHROPLASTY FOR DIGITAL DEFORMITIES

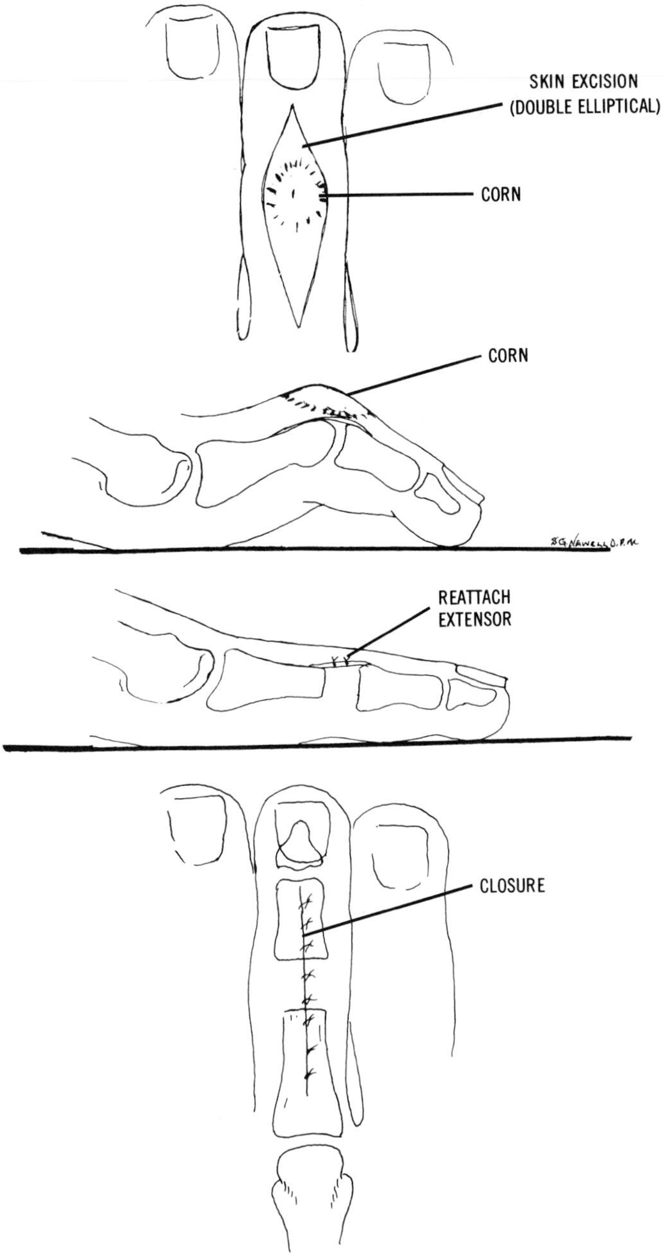

Hallux Valgus With Bunion Deformities

The young athlete with painful hallux valgus with bunion deformity is afforded the most sophisticated surgical procedures available. In such a manner, osteotomies are commonly used to correct bony deformities of either the first metatarsal or proximal phalanx. These are done in conjunction with arthroplasty procedures of the first metatarsal phalangeal joint. All attempts are made to salvage the joint while realigning both the proximal and the distal set angles (Figures 10-15).[9]

FIGURE 10

X RAY AP VIEW OF FEET PREOPERATIVE

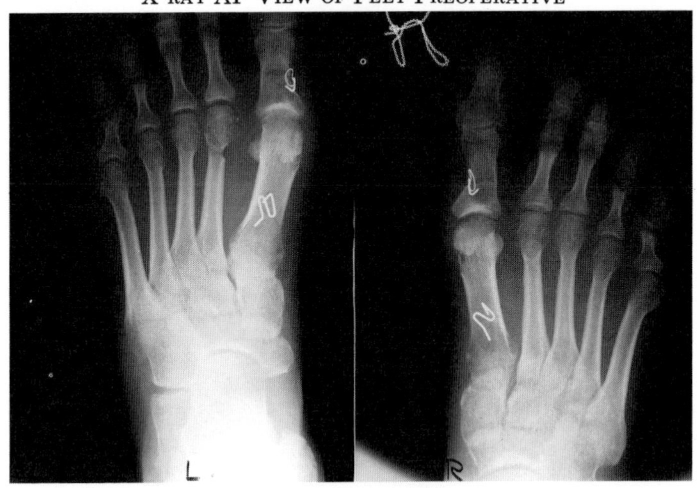

FIGURE 11

X RAY AP VIEW OF FEET POSTOPERATIVE

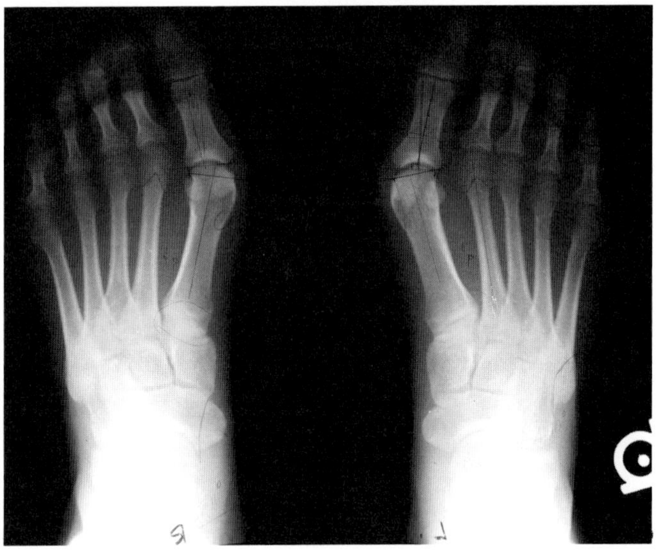

FIGURE 12
X RAY PATIENT N.S. PREOPERATIVE
ANTERIOR POSTERIOR VIEW

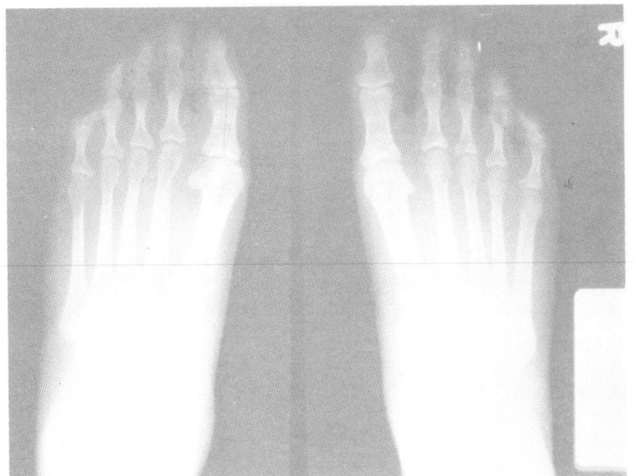

Bilateral hallux valgus with long second metatarsals. Prominent styloid fifth metatarsal left and os navicularis right. Both fourth and fifth toes are contracted.

FIGURE 13
POSTOPERATIVE ANTERIOR POSTERIOR
VIEW PATIENT FOLLOWING AIKEN PROCEDURE
LEFT GREAT TOE

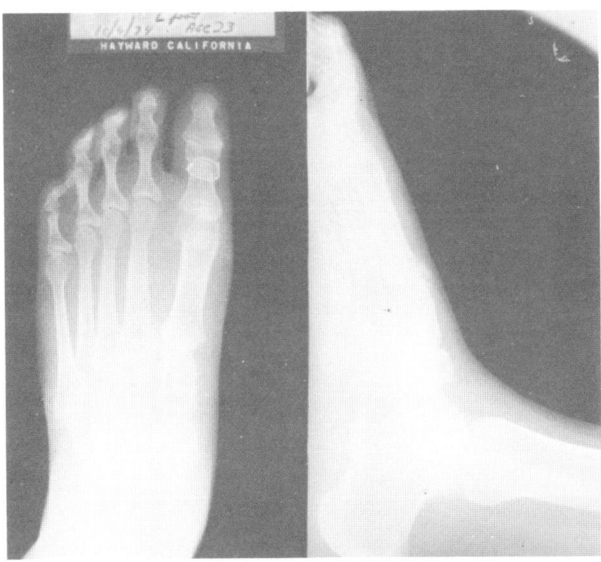

When arthritic deformities are present, a resection implant arthroplastry is carried out. A Swanson Silastic implant is utilized with care being taken to save the intrinsic muscular attachments to the proximal phalanx (Figure 15). In cases where this has been carried out, the success rate is excellent. These athletes are able to return to competition within two months following the surgical procedures.[10]

FIGURE 14
OSTEOTOMIES TO CORRECT METATARSUS PRIMUS ADDUCTOS WITH HALLUX VALGUS

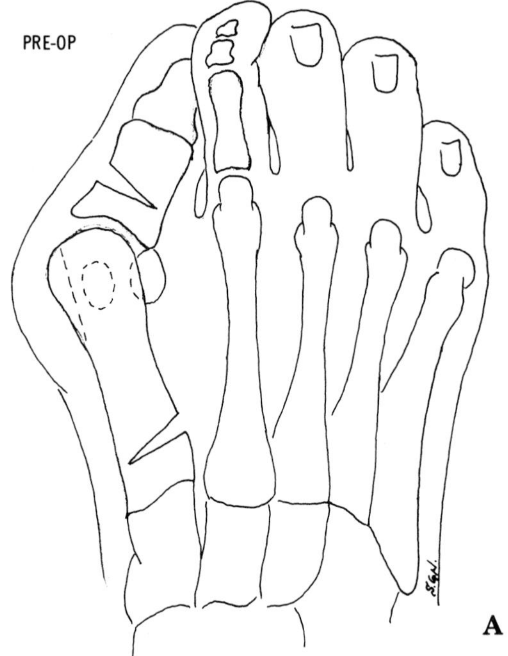

CLOSING WEDGE — AIKEN MCBRIDE PROCEDURE:

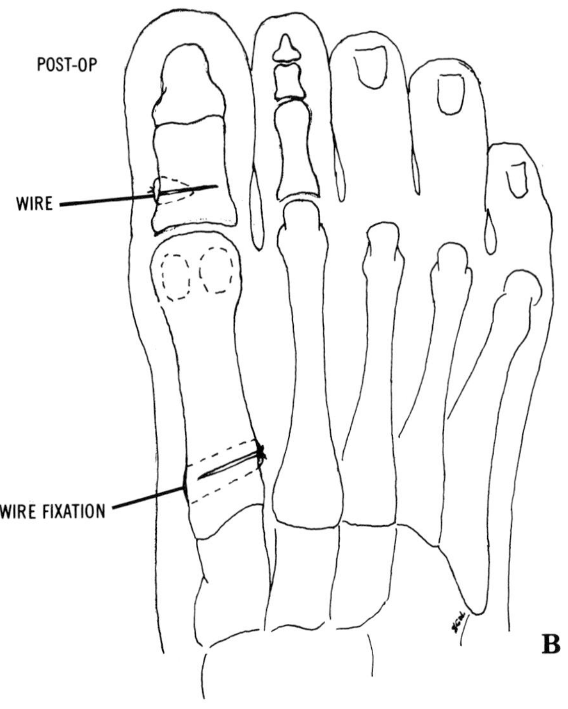

FIGURE 15A
Preoperative Hallux Limitus

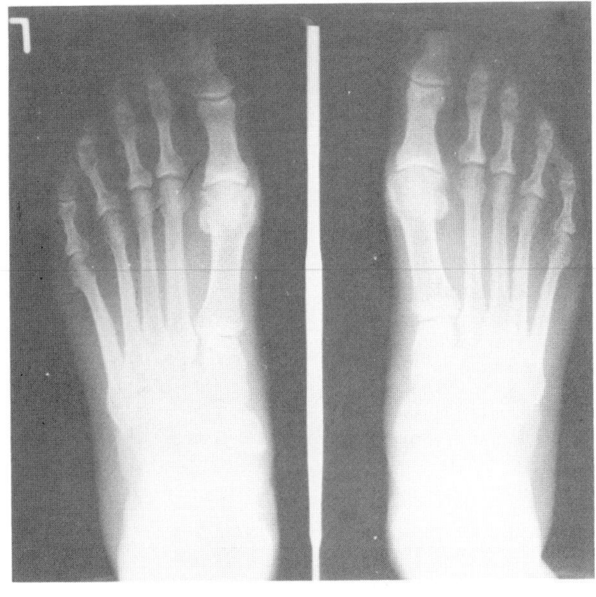

FIGURE 15B
Postoperative Implant Arthroplasty with
First Metatarsal Head Remodeling

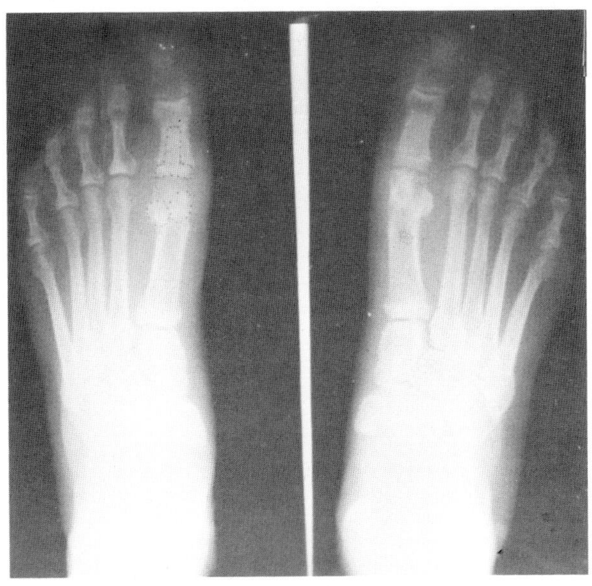

Tailor's Bunionette

When marked splaying of the fifth metatarsal is present I prefer an osteotomy to reduce the deformity. In this way, I preserve the fifth metatarsal phalangeal joint.[11] It may be neccessary also to do a partial osteotomy of a prominent bony projection of the fifth metatarsal head with this procedure (Figures 16 and 17). In cases where the fifth metatarsal is both abducted and plantar flexed, a biplane osteotomy is performed.[11] In cases where the fifth metatarsal is in relatively good alignment, but yet an exostosis still exists, a partial osteotomy in a closed manner is carried out with good results.

The osteotomies require casting for six weeks in a below-the-knee walking cast. During this time the athlete may ride a bike or exercise in other ways which will not damage the cast itself. In the older athletes with a fifth metatarsal head problem, a partial resection of the fifth metatarsal head is carried out in such a manner that extreme shortening will not occur. We call this a hemi-head resection.[9]

FIGURE 16
Closing Wedge Osteotomy Fifth Metatarsal

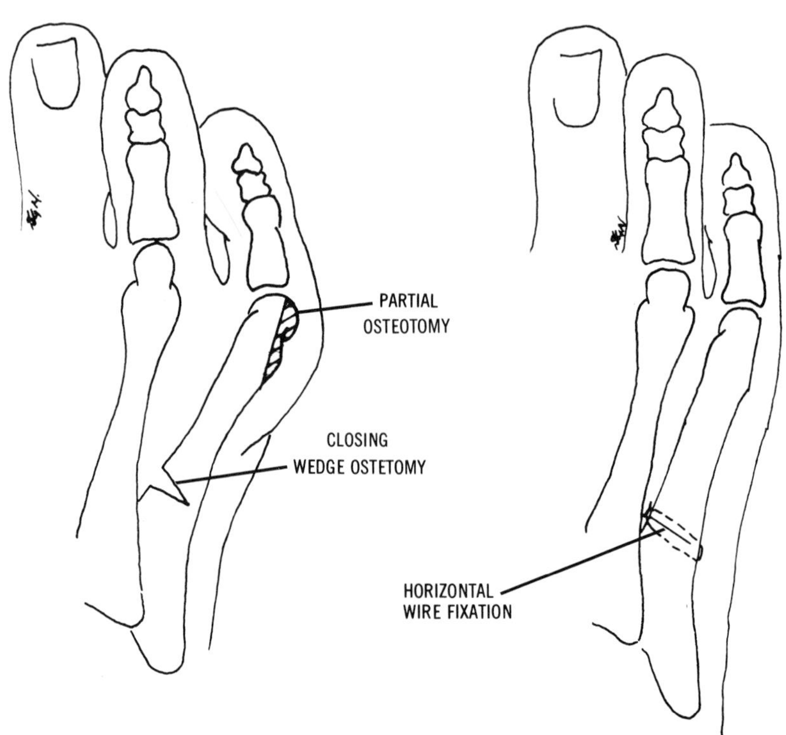

FIGURE 17A

Preoperative Foot with Tailor's
Bunion B Left and Hallux Valgus Right

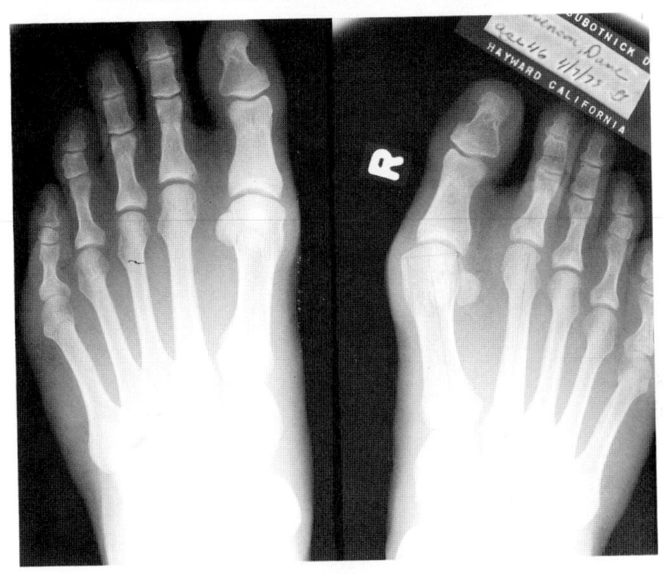

FIGURE 17B

Postoperative McBride Bunion Procedure
and Partial Ostectomies for Taylor's Bunionettes

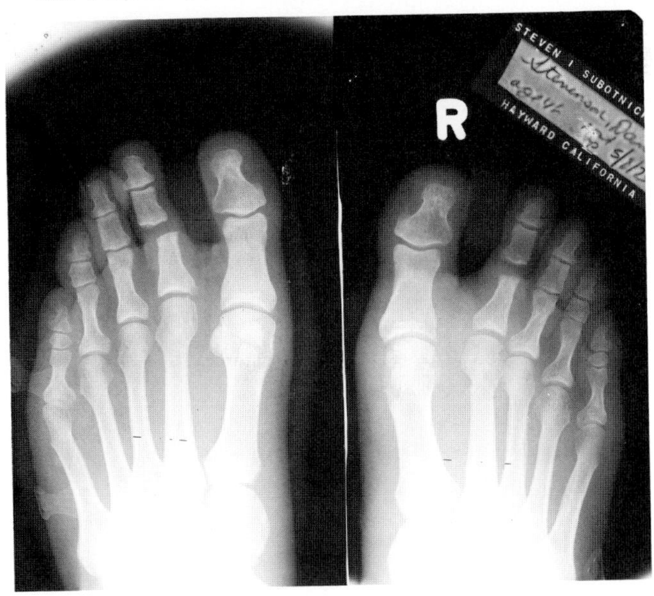

Plantar Keratomas

Intractable plantar keratomas secondary to plantar positioning of a metatarsal head which fails to respond to neutral control are best treated by dorsal osteotomies of the involved metatarsals (Figure 18).[36] When a rigid foot type is present we prefer to do a dorsal closing wedge osteotomy near the metatarsal base (Figure 19).[10] This osteotomy generally requires a two millimeter wedge with the base of the wedge dorsal. An incomplete fracture is carried out and the osteotomy is closed with a wire fixation (Figure 11). When central metatarsals are involved it is generally permissable to utilize a below-the-ankle walking cast for six weeks to allow for proper healing. When the first metatarsal head is involved, then a below-the-knee walking cast is utilized for six weeks.

FIGURE 18
WEDGE OSTEOTOMIES

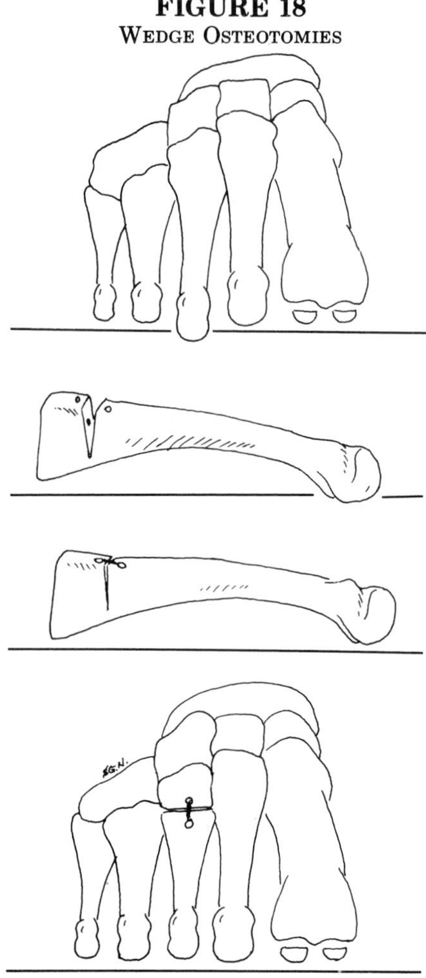

FIGURE 19

AXIAL VIEW OF FOOT

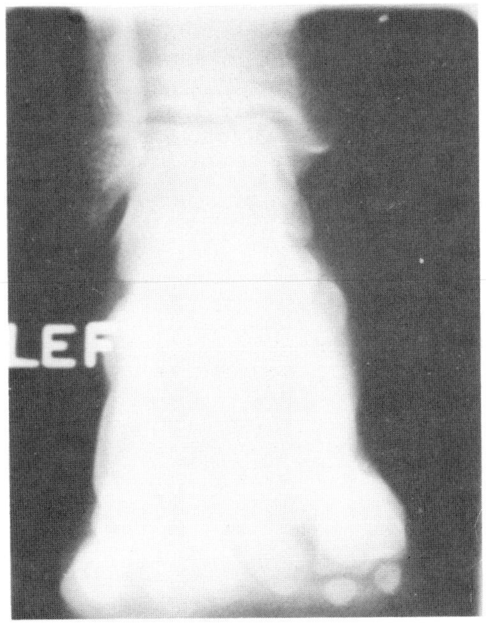

FIGURE 20

AP VIEW OF BASKETBALL PLAYERS FEET WITH ADVANCED BUNIONS. NOTE LONG SECOND METATARSALS AND "SPLAY" FEET

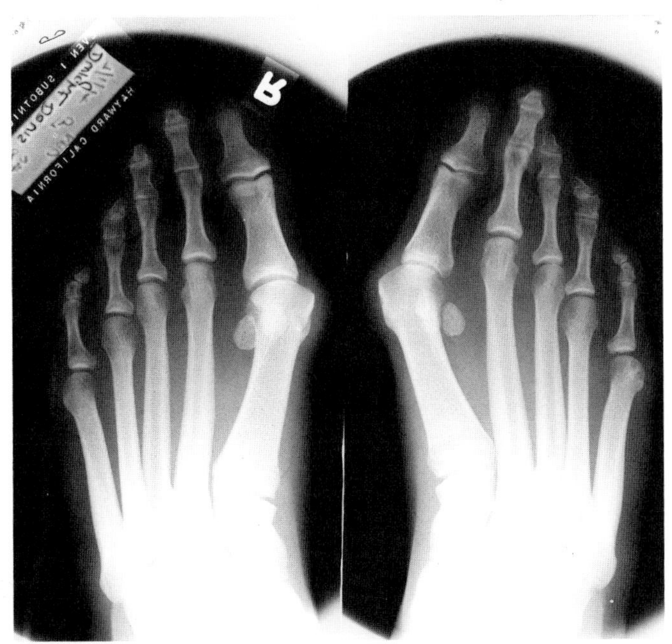

For isolated plantar keratomas in a more mobile foot, we have had good success utilizing a V-osteotomy carried out between the surgical anatomical necks of the metatarsal[10] (Figures 20,21,22). These osteotomies need no internal fixations or external casting.

FIGURE 21

POSTOPERATIVE X RAYS

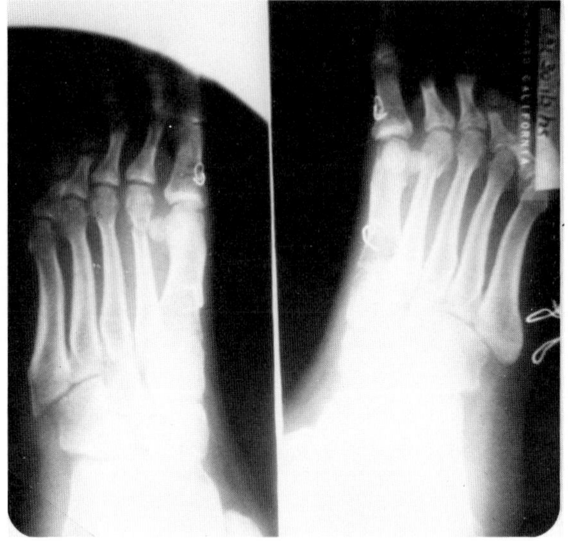

Dorsal wedge osteotomies first metatarsals, removal medial cuneiform exostosis "R", remodeling of styloid process fifth "L".

FIGURE 22

(V) OSTEOTOMIES

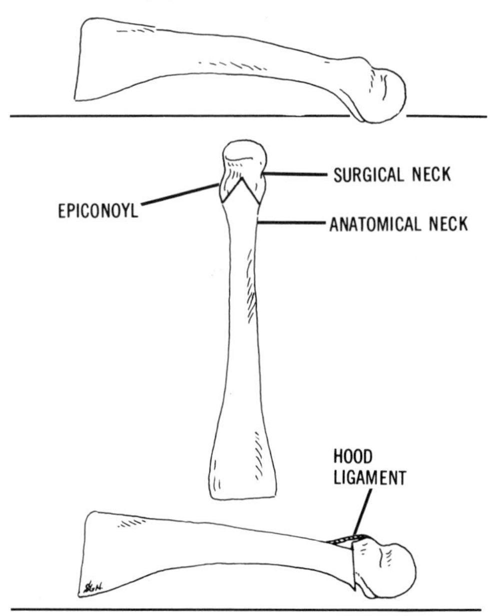

It is important that this osteotomy is done with the apex of the "V" being distal and at the surgical neck of the metatarsal. In this way, the soft tissue structures comprising the hood extensor apparatus stablize the osteotomy. Following this surgical procedure, the patient is maintained in a wooden postoperative shoe for three to four weeks. Between the third and fifth week, there is generally some dorsal swelling in this area as the fracture is healing. This may be tender. The athlete is not allowed to return to full activity for six weeks. It is to be noted that these intractable keratomas generally occur in the older athletes.

Calcaneal Planter Spurs

Calcaneal plantar spurs are generally symptomatic following chronic abuse. When conservative treatment has failed, it may be necessary to surgically excise the radiographic present spur and release the plantar fascia as well as the first layer of the plantar intrinsic muscles.[8] This procedure is best carried out under a dry field through a medial longitudinal skin incision at the junction of the thick and thin skin. A long incision is necessary to adequately visualize the spur. The spur is localized by blunt and sharp dissection and, following the removal of the soft tissue from the spur, it is excised with an osteotome and mallet. It is equally important when carrying out this procedure to release the plantar fascia as it is to remove the calcaneal spur. When the possibility of a plantar neuroma is present, it should be excised from its location in the plantar fat pad (Figure 23). Likewise, an adventitious bursitis should be surgically removed (Figures 2 and 4, Chapter 15). Heel spur surgery will prevent normal activity for two to three months. The soft tissue is generally healed well within four weeks, but reorganization takes place for quite some time. The only restricting factor in returning to normal activity is the pain itself following this surgical procedure. It is to be noted that this surgical procedure is an end result of exhaustive attempts at conservative treatment which more times than not are successful.

FIGURE 23
Calcaneal Spurs and Retrocalcaneal Exostosis

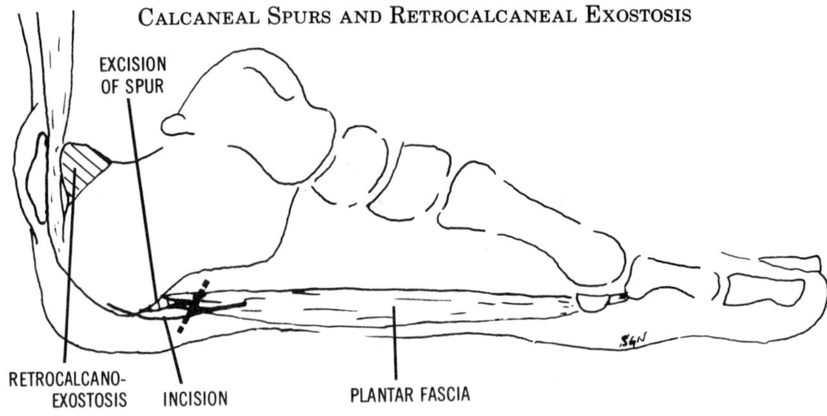

FIGURE 24
Retrocalcaneal Exostosis

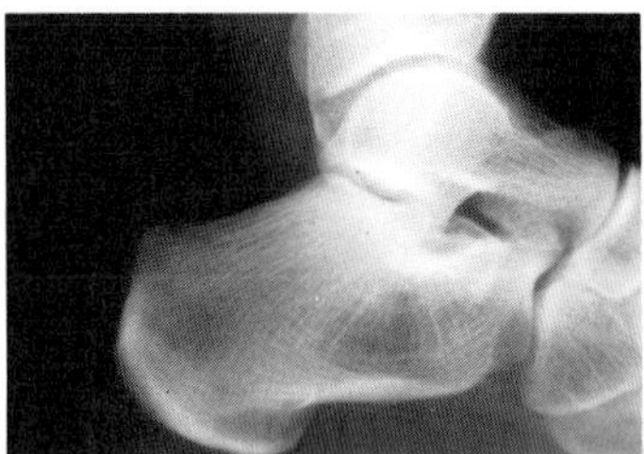

A. Preoperative

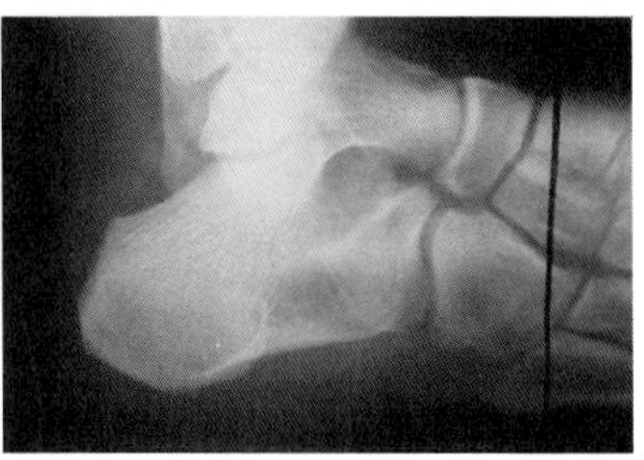

B. Postoperative

Retro-Calcaneal Exostosis

The retrocalcaneal exostosis which is refractory to conservative treatment is best treated by surgical excision.[8,40] The incision which we now utilize is a transverse approach carried out in a skin line over the attachment of tendo Achillis to the superior aspect of the posterior surface of the calcaneus (Figures 20,21,24,25). Through this incision, it is generally easy to localize the hyperostotic aspects of the bone across the whole superior posterior aspect of the distal one third of the calcaneus (Figures 9, 22,23). The tendo Achillis is gently retracted and freed from the superior one-third posterior surface of the calcaneus and this aspect of the bone is then resected with a bone-cutting instrument. It may be necessary to partially free the tendo Achillis from its attachments into the middle one third of the calcaneus if soft tissue damage secondary to bony hypertrophy has been present in this area. Care should be taken in resecting bone in this area. The raw bone surface should be well smoothed and adequate flushing of the wound carried out. The tendo Achillis should be treated gently and its superior surface should be inspected and adventitious bursitis resected. Adhesions at the area of paratenon of the superior surface of the tendo Achillis may be freed by soft tissue dissection. This should be carried out bluntly. Following the surgical procedures the tissue is closed in layers and a moderate compressive dressing is applied. A below-the-knee cast with the foot 90 degrees to the leg is applied with a walker. This cast is maintained for three to four weeks during which isometric and isotonic exercises are carried out. Following removal of the cast, the patient returns to normal activity with pain and stiffness being the main limiting factor. There are various amounts of postoperative edema following this procedure but there may be less with the transverse approach, than with the traditional longitudinal skin incision at the lateral aspect of the tendo Achillis. When extensive paratenosis damage is anticipated, a longitudinal incision affords better access (Figures 23,24).

FIGURE 25A

Preoperative Talar Neck Exostosis

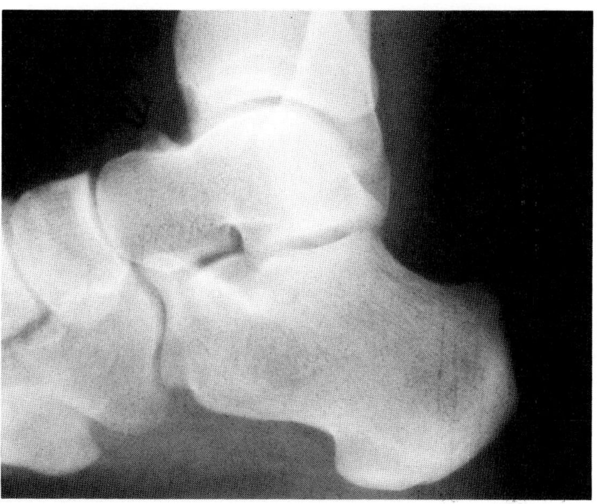

FIGURE 25B
POSTOPERATIVE TALAR NECK EXOSTOSIS

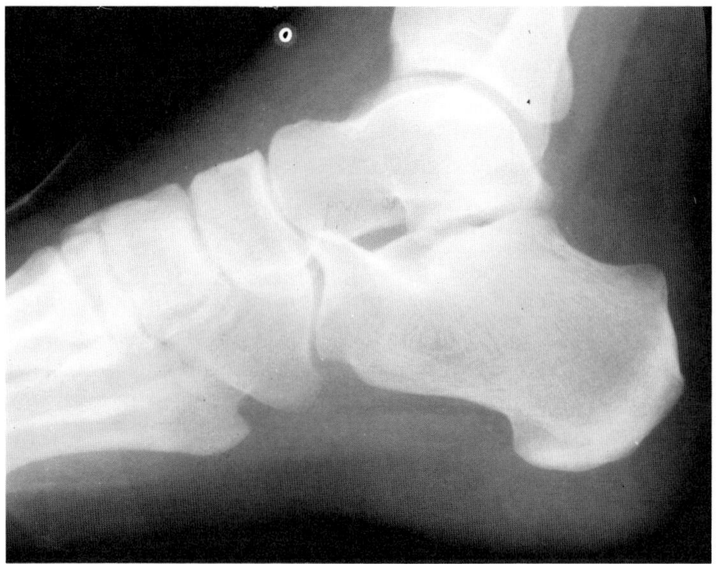

Talar Exostosis

The anterior talar neck impingement exostosis which may be complicated by an exostosis also of the tibia at the anterior aspect of the ankle joint, is treated by surgical excision when pain is present or when functional limitations at the ankle joint are present. The isolated exostosis of the talar neck may occur with a compression of the neurovascular bundles in this area. A release of neurovascular bundles and then excision of the hypertrophic bone is carried out through a dorsal longitudinal skin incision. When an impingement exostosis between the tibia and the talus is present this is best treated through a dorsal longitudinal skin incision placed over the neurovascular bundle. The tissue layers are resected with retraction utilizing black silk suture of the various layers. In this manner the extensor retinaculum is isolated and freed as are the superficial nerves and deep nerves and vessels. The anterior distal aspect of the tibia when involved with the impingement exostosis appears pink and somewhat arthritic. This abnormal bone is resected with care being taken not to disrupt the superior talar dome. The excessive bone on the talar neck is likewise resected to allow for a normal configuration and normal dorsiflexion. Following this procedure the tendo Achillis may be tight, but this will gradually stretch out with proper physical therapy carried out postoperatively. Closure, following adequate flushing of the wound, is done in layers and in these cases the extensor retinaculum may be loosely approximated. The patient is maintained in a below-the-knee nonweight-bearing cast for four weeks followed by a below-the-knee weight-bearing cast for an additional four weeks. When more extensive dissection of bone is carried out, it may be necessary to utilize plaster mobilization for a total of ten weeks. When isolated talar neck exostosis are resected, a below-the-knee walking cast is used for between three to four weeks.

Os Trigonum and Posterior Talar Shelves

The symtomatic os trigonum or posterior talar shelves is resected through a curvalinear longitudinal lateral approach. This incision is placed just behind the lateral malleolus. Care is taken to isolate the sural nerve, as well as the peroneal tendons during the dissection of the soft tissue. The os trigonum itself is somewhat difficult to locate in its deep location at the heel aspect. It is free from its soft tissue attachments which often times include the posterior lateral collateral ligament of the ankle joint. It is then carefully dissected free and any protruding posterior talar shelve is resected. The isolated posterior talar shelve is visualized through a similar incision and resected with a bone cutting instrument. Arthritic calcaneus bone is resected. Following adequate wound flushing and soft tissue closure, the patient is maintained in a below-the-knee nonweight-bearing cast for two to three weeks following which a walking heel is applied and the cast maintained for an additional three weeks. This allows for adequate soft tissue healing about the subtalar joint. Following the removal of the cast, range of motion exercises are utilized and the athlete may return to normal activity when full range of motion is achieved. These procedures generally preclude normal activity for periods of up to two to three months (Figures 26,27,28).

FIGURE 26
EXTENSION OF TALAR POSTERIOR PROCESS BEYOND SUBTALAR JOINT.
PREOPERATIVE OS TRIGONUM

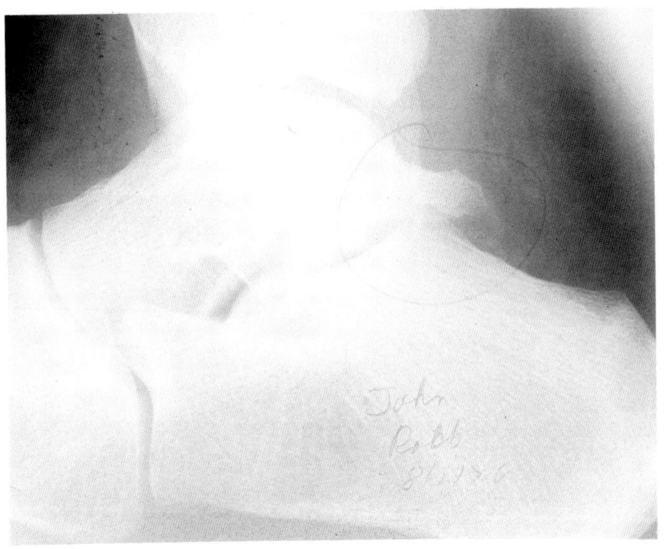

Extension of talar posterior process beyond subtalar joint.

FIGURE 27
REMOVAL OF OS TRIGONUM

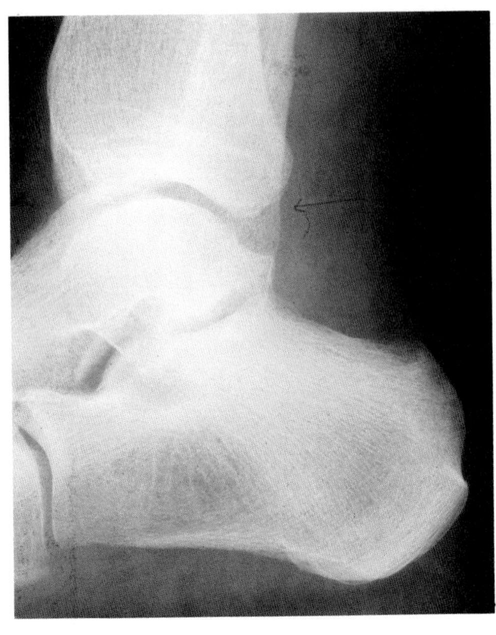

Removal of os trigonum

FIGURE 28
IMPINGEMENT EXOSTOSIS — ANTERIOR ANKLE WITH POSTFRACTURE ARTHRITIC POSTERIOR STJ SHELF

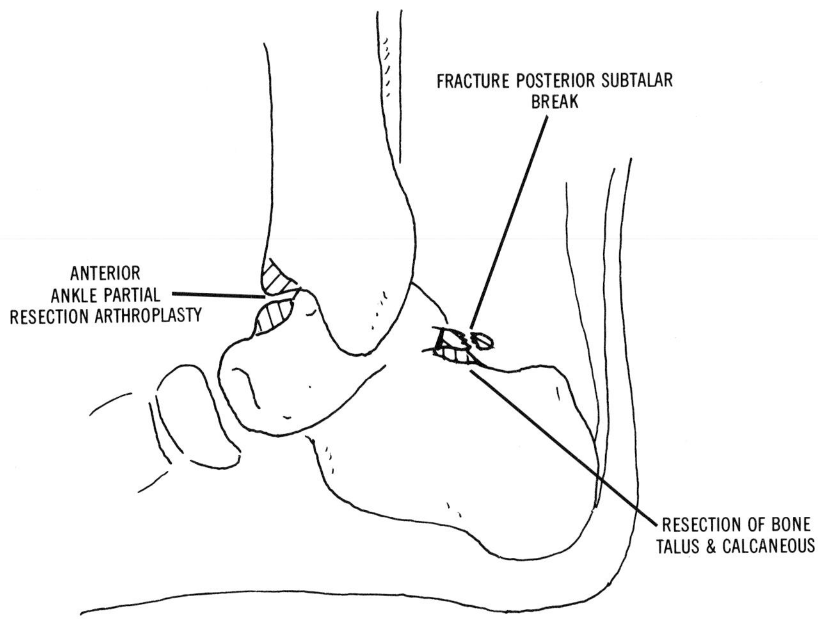

FIGURE 29
OS NAVICULARUS

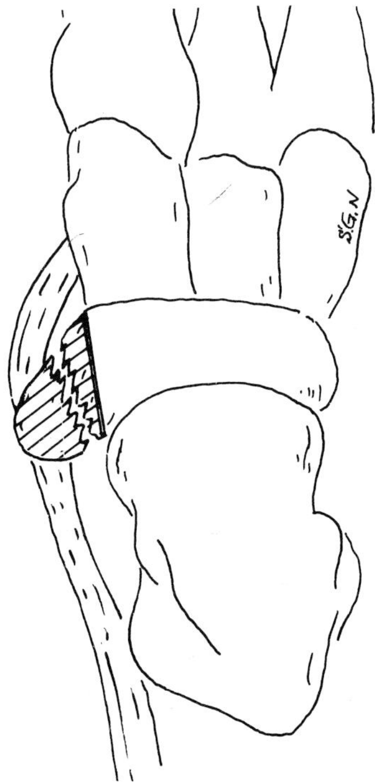

Os Navicularis

The os navicularis is generally excised through a medial dorsal longitudinal skin incision (Figure 29).[33] Care is taken to free the posterior tibial tendon from the protruding tubercle of the navicular when a separate center of ossification is not present (Figure 30). When a true second ossicle is present, the posterior tibial tendon is isolated and retracted properly and then the medial protuberance of the navicular is resected flush to the medial surface of the first cuneiform. Care is taken not to damage the head of the talus. Following this, it is easy to excise the ossicle from the attachments of the posterior tibial tendon. When doing this procedure on a younger child with a flatfoot deformity, transpose the posterior tibial tendon plantarly. When doing this procedure on an older individual, the posterior tibial tendon is merely placed in a proper anatomical position and no attempt to stabilize it with soft tissue is carried out. I have found that the soft tissue repositioning of the tendon with a retinaculoplasty in the adult precludes a posterior tibial tendonitis which may prolong the rehabilitative course. The patient utilizes the below-the-knee walking cast for four weeks following the surgical procedures to allow for proper healing and positioning of the posterior tibial tendon. The athletes return to normal activity between eight to ten weeks following the surgical procedure.

FIGURE 30

Os Navicularis

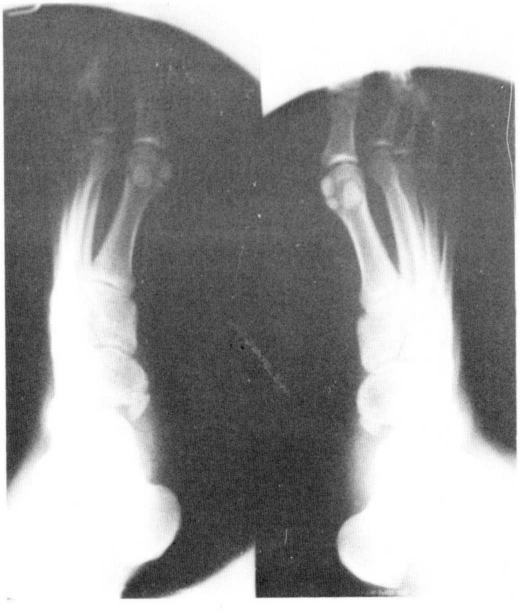

SUMMARY

I have presented those soft tissue and bony deformities which are more prevalent among athletes and have suggested possible surgical approaches for these problems. I feel that optimal surgical results should be planned for and that adequate postoperative splinting or casting should be used. It is possible for the athlete to continue some form of training utilizing isometric and isotonic exercises with proper immobilization of the part which was operated on. The athletes may walk or ride a bike with plaster paris casts on. Likewise, they may do range of motion exercises of the nonstabilized parts. Surgery may often times be the most conservative approach for foot problems. When carefully planned surgical procedures are carried out, the results are expected to be good.

Bibliography

1. American Academy of Orthopedic Surgeons, "Symposium on Sports Medicine", C.V. Mosby Co., St. Louis, 1969.
2. Blazina, M.E., Kerlan, R.K., Jobe, F.W., Carter, V.S., Carlson, Joanne G., *Jumper's Knee,* Orthopedic Clinics of Northern America, Vol. 4, No. 3: 665-678, July 1973.
3. Brubaker, T.E., James, S.L., *Injuries to Runners,* Laboratory for Human Performance, University of Oregon, 1974.
4. Cerney, J.P., *Complete Book of Athletic Taping Techniques,* Parker Publishing Incorp., West Nyak, N.Y.
5. Corrigan, A.B. and Fitch, K.E., "Complications of Jogging", *The Medical Journal of Australia,* 363, 1972.
6. Craig, T.T., *Comments in Sports Medicine, JAMA,* 231: 333, 1973.
7. DuVries, H.L., *Physiology of Exercises for Physical Education and Athletics,* William Brown & Company, 1966.
8. DuVries, H.L., *Surgery of the Foot,* C.V. Mosby Co., St. Louis, 1964.
9. Gerbert, J. et al, *The Surgical Treatment of the Intractable Plantar Keratoma,* Futura Publishing Company, Mt. Kisco, N.Y., 247 pp.
10. Gerbert, J., Mercado, O.A., Sokoloff, T.H., *The Surgical Treatment of the Hallux-Abducto-Valgus and Allied Deformities,* Futura Publishing Company, Mt. Kisco, N.Y., 140 pp.
11. Gerbert, J., Sgarlato, T.E., and Subotnick, S.I., Preliminary Study of a Closing Wedge Osteotomy of the Fifth Metatarsal for Correction of Tailor's Bunion Deformity, *JAPA* 62:212-218, 1972.
12. Jackson, D.W., and Bailey, D., Shin Splints in the Young White: A Non-Specific Diagnosis, *The Physician and Sports Medicine,* Vol. 3, No. 3: 45-51, 1975.
13. James, S.L., and Brubaker, C.E., "Biomechanics of Running", *Orthopedics of America,* Vol. 4, No. 3: 605-616, July 1973.
14. James, S.L., Personal Communication. 1975.
15. Johnson and Johnson, *Therapeutic Uses of Adhesive Tape,* Second Edition, New Brunswick, N.J. 1958.
16. Kline, C., Alman, F.L., Jr., *The Knee in Sports,* Jenkins Publishing Company, The Premerton Press, Austin, Texas.
17. McGlamary, E.D., Gastrocnemius Tendon Recession, *JAPA,* 3:163.
18. Nellen, J.W., *Medicine and the Green Bay Packers,* Upjohn Company, 1968.
19. Nicholas, J.A., Injuries to the Menisci of the Knee. *Orthopedic Clinic North America,* Vol. 4, No. 3: 647-664, 1975.
20. O'Donoghue, D.H., Treatment of Acute Ligamentous Injuries of the Knee. *Orthopedic Clinic North America,* Vol. 4, No. 3:617-645, 1975.
21. O'Donoghue, D.H., *Treatment of Injuries to Athletes,* Second Edition, W.B. Saunders Company, Philadelphia, 1970.
22. Root, M.L., Orien, W., Weed, J.H., Hughs, R.J., *Biomechanical Examination of the Foot,* Vol. l, Clinical Biomechanics Corp., Los Angeles, 1971.
23. Sgarlato, T.E., *A Compendium of Podiatric Biomechanics,* California College of Podiatric Medicine, 1971.
24. Sheehan, G.M., Chondromalacia in Runners, *Amer. College of Sports Medicine Newsletter,* Vol. 7, No. 4, 1972.
25. Sheehan, G.M., Encyclopedia Athletic Medicine, *Runner's World Booklet of the Month,* No. 12, 1972.
26. Sherman, H.M., The Operative Treatment of Pes Cavus, *American Journal Orthopedic Surgeons,* 2:374-380, 1965.
27. Slocum, D.B., James, S.L., Biomechanics of Running, *JAMA,* Vol. 205, No. ll: 97-104, September 9, 1968.

28. Slocum, D.B., Larson, R.L., James, S.L., Late Reconstruction Procedures Used to Stabilize the Knee, *Orthopedic Clinic North America,* Vol. 4, No.3:679-689, 1975.
29. Subotnick, S.I., editor, *Athlete's Feet,* Runner's World Publications.
30. Subotnick, S.I., The Biomechanical Basis of Skiing, *JAPA,* 1:54-66, 1974.
31. Subotnick, S.I., Compartment Syndromes in The Lower Extremities, *JAPA,* 65,4:342-347, 1975.
32. Subotnick, S.I., The Equinus Deformity as it Effects the Forefoot, *JAPA,* 61:423-427, 1971.
33. Subotnick, S.I., The Flexible Flatfoot, *Archives of Podiatric Medicine and Foot Surgery,* Vol. 1, No. 1: 7-33, 1973.
34. Subotnick, S.I., Long Legs, Short Legs, *Runner's World,* Vol. 9: 21-22, March 1974.
35. Subotnick, S.I., Morton's Foot, *Runner's World,* Vol. 94, April 1974.
36. Subotnick, S.I., Observations of Plantar Callouses, *Archives of Podiatric Medicine and Foot Surgery,* Vol. 1, No. 4: 329-337.
37. Subotnick, S.I., Orthotic Foot Control in the Overuse Syndrome, *The Physician in Sports Medicine,* Vol. 3, No.1: 75-79, January 1975.
38. Subotnick, S.I., The Overuse Syndrome of the Foot and Leg, Part II, California College of Podiatric Medicine, April 1974.
39. Subotnick, S.I., Shoes and Injuries in Shoes for Runners, *Runner's World Booklet of the Month,* No. 25: 70-71, July 1973.
40. Subotnick, S.I., Why Bumps Grow, *Runner's World Magazine,* March 1973, 24-30.

Appendix 1

Compartment Syndromes in the Lower Extremities

STEVEN I. SUBOTNICK, D.P.M.*

After a brief discussion of the normal anatomy of the leg, the pathophysiology and clinical features of the compartment syndrome are presented. The various etiologies of the compartment syndrome are then discussed in detail. The primary etiologic factor appears to be a loss of microcirculation to the muscles. This decrease in microcirculation can be caused by 1) strenuous muscular activity, 2) fractures, sprains and contusions or 3) vascular injuries and diseases. The treatment of the compartment syndrome is discussed. The importance of differentiating between the exercise idiopathic form of compartment syndrome and shin splints and strains is stressed. It is also stressed that prompt surgical fasciotomy will considerably lessen the incidence of disability following the compartment syndrome.

The leg presents with three well defined compartments which are non-yielding in character and are prone to produce ischemic damage to muscle and nerves when intractable swelling is present. Although the anterior compartment is most frequently involved in the compartment syndrome, the lateral and posterior compartments may also be involved under varying circumstances ranging from athletic overuse of muscles to direct contusion (1—7). Since the disability from the compartment syndrome appears to be preventable by early recognition and treatment, a review of the present knowledge appears to be proper (2).

Anatomical Considerations

The lower leg is divided into three fascial compartments. The fascia is firmly attached proximally at the knee, and distally it is strengthened about the ankle by three sets of retinacula (Fig. 1). The interosseous membrane divides the leg into the anterior and posterior compartments. Additionally, two deep septa attach to the fibula over the lateral aspect of the leg and form a lateral compartment. Except for perforation of the fascia by blood vessels and nerves, and the exit of tendons distally, these compartments are essentially closed spaces (8). The posterior muscular compartment may be further divided into the posterior deep and the posterior superficial compartment.

The blood supply into the muscles of the anterior or extensor compartment is chiefly from the anterior tibial artery. The anterior tibial muscle receives almost all of its supply from the anterior tibial vessel, whereas the

* Assistant Professor of Surgery and Biomechanics, California College of Podiatric Medicine, and Co-Chief, Foot Clinic, San Francisco General Hospital

extensor digitorum longus and the extensor hallucis longus receive additional perforating branches from the peroneal and from the posterior tibial artery. The peroneal vessels supply the lateral compartment (peroneal) muscles and the posterior tibial vessels the posterior compartment (flexor) muscles. The intramuscular vascular pattern is an important factor in the susceptibility of a particular muscle to ischemia. The gastrocnemius muscle is sensitive to any interruption of its blood supply because it lacks the intramuscular anastomoses (8).

The deep peroneal nerve supplies the muscles of the anterior compartment. The lateral compartment musculature is innervated by the superficial peroneal nerve and the posterior compartment by the posterior tibial nerve.

Pathophysiology

The lower leg consists of three relatively unyielding fascial compartments, each supplied by one major vessel and nerve.

Lueck and Ray (8) point out that in the major vessels of the leg the arterial pressure is approximately 100 mm Hg; as the arteries branch into arterioles the pressure falls to about 40 mm. Hg. The pressure at the capillary level is between 20 and 30 mm. Hg. At the venous level the pressure has been measured 10 to 15 mm. Hg (Fig. 2).

Skeletal muscle is able to produce energy during periods of anoxia by the anaerobic cycle. This creates an oxygen debt which is replenished later by local factors which increase local blood flow. However, if this is not replaced a high concentration of lactic acid and anoxia may lead to muscle necrosis (8).

It would appear that any condition which raises the intrafascial pressure about 15 to 40 mm. Hg will effectively block the blood supply to the muscles without necessarily occluding the major arteries, which have a higher pressure gradient (9). It is possible to develop compartment ischemia without interrupting the dorsalis pedis or posterior tibial pulses (10).

Figure 1. Cross section of leg.

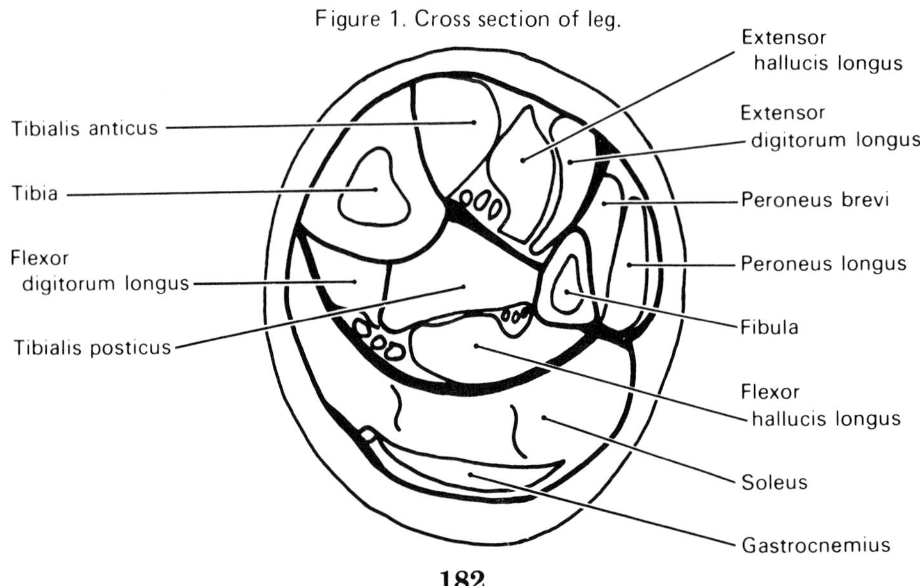

Appendix 1

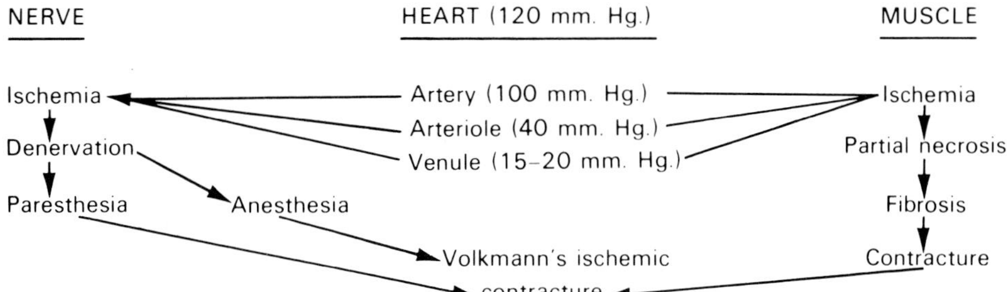

Figure 2. Postulated sequence of events producing Volkmann's ischemic contracture (from Lueck, R. A. and Ray, R. D.: Volkmann's ischemia of the lower extremity. Surg. Clin. North Am., 52: 145, 1972.).

Clinical Features

Classically, the compartment syndrome has been in reference to the anterior compartment of the leg. The symptoms are pain, pallor, paresthesias, pulselessness and, finally, paralysis. These symptoms, in the case of the anterior tibial compartment syndrome, may be absent with the only symptom present being that of firmness over the fascial compartment and painful movement with severe pain which gradually worsens. The overlying skin is reddened, glossy, and warm, and soon a "woody tension" develops. There is severe pain out of proportion to the injury and loss of function becomes evident with progression of the compartment syndrome (7). Early muscle damage occurs within 4 to 6 hr and irreversible changes occur within 18 hr. Painful movement, severe pain which gradually worsens, hypesthesia in the area supplied by the peripheral nerves, and weakness hypesthesia in the area supplied by the peripheral nerves, and weakness or paralysis are commonly associated with this condition (11). Carter (10) reported upon nine cases of anterior compartment syndrome with palpable anterior pulses. French and Prince (12) reported a compartment syndrome which presents with moderate to severe pain in the anterior compartment after exercise, without frank foot drop, with symptoms as long as 5 years before medical attention was sought. These symptoms were relieved by fasciotomy.

Etiologies

A wide variety of injuries may lead to the disastrous end results of the compartment syndrome, Volkmann's contracture. All of these share some loss of blood supply to the effected muscles (8). Crush injuries, tibial fractures and ischemic contracture following the use of braces have been reported (2-4, 6, 12-16). There have also been reports of Volkmann's ischemic contracture following vascular disease and vascular leakage (17—20). Benjamin (21) and Holmes (22) comment upon ischemic nerve damage. Gardner (23) reported a compartment syndrome in the arm secondary to minor trauma in the hand. He concluded that the compartment syndrome was the direct result of a reflex arch arterial spasm. Critchley (4) reported on the increase of bulk on fatigued muscles. Lewis (9) reported upon the effect of increased tissue pressure which resulted in decreased tissue perfusion. Parkes (24) also reported upon the ischemic effects of pressure. Scherr and his associates (25) reported upon loss of tissue viability as demonstrated by the doppler. Wolfort (11) reported upon compartment syndromes following fascial herniation repair. All agreed that intractable pressure is the etiologic factor in compartment syndromes, regardless of the cause.

Bradley (2) prefers to group the various etiologies of compartment syndromes into three basic groups. Group 1 is that of the "idiopathic exercise" form following strenous muscular activity. Group 2 is that of the traumatic compartment syndrome following fractures, sprains and contusions. Group 3 is that of the vascular etiology compartment syndromes following vascular injuries, diseases and thromboembolism. Bradley refers to 137 cases reported with acute anterior compartment syndrome. Forty-five of these cases fell into Group 1, 26 into Group 2 and 52 in Group 3. Of the patients in this series, 95% were male. All patients had symptoms of pain, swelling and tenderness. Of the patients with anterior compartment syndrome, 72% had hypesthesia at the dorsal aspect of the first web space of the foot. The dorsalis pedis pulse was present in the majority of the non-vascular cases. Fasciotomy carried out before foot drop occurred resulted in complete recovery. Fasciotomy carried out after foot drop occurred resulted in 13% complete recovery.

Group I. Idiopathic Compartment Syndrome Etiologies. In this group there is a history of severe unaccustomed exercise. This occurs most frequently in the male around the age of 23 years. The right leg is affected twice as much as the left leg. The dorsalis pedis remains normal in 75% of these patients, with hypesthesia at the dorsal aspect of the first web being present in 65% of the patients. The etiology for group 1-type compartment syndromes would be that of increased tissue pressure following unaccustomed exercise. There is a decreased arterial perfusion and a relative muscle ischemia. An additional factor may be muscular strains with secondary bleeding into the closed compartment's space (6). The exercise form of compartment syndrome appears to be reversible because the condition is gradual. With pain, the athlete should stop exercise, rest, have his limb elevated and packed in ice, and be observed (3, 6). This form of idiopathic compartment syndrome is also seen in the lateral compartment (1) and has been reported in the posterior compartment (4). These symptoms of localized severe pain which increase with range of motion must be differentiated from shin splints (26). Shin splints may occur in the anterior compartment secondary to heel contact on hard surfaces or biomechanical abnormalities such as forefoot varus. The author has observed that in these cases the anterior tibial muscle works overtime in its efforts to decelerate the foot at contact and stabilize the foot when excessive varus deformity is present. Shin splints may be the result of partial avulsion of the muscles from the attachments to the tibia, fibula and interosseous membranes. Shin splints may also be present in the posterior (flexor) compartment, which is appreciated more often during toe off.

Group 1 idiopathic compartment syndrome must also be differentiated from strains which are partial ruptures of the muscle tendon units (3). These can occur with overuse of the motor units in the conditioned athlete as well as overstress of the motor units in the unconditioned athlete. Overuse injuries are usually those of the chronic repetitive strain and the overstress injuries are those of the acute strain such as that seen in a sprinter coming out of the starting blocks. Both shin splints and strain respond well to elevation and immediate application of ice and the tenderness and firmness does not progress. With progression of firmness and pain a form of group 1 idiopathic compartment syndrome may be occurring. Patients must be watched very carefully and at the first sign of true compartment syndrome non-responsive to local treatment a fasciotomy must be carried out (2, 3, 6, 27).

It is interesting to note that the idiopathic form of compartment syndrome presents most commonly with involvement of the extensor hallucis longus muscle, followed by the anterior tibial muscle and lastly by the extensor digitorum longus muscles. It is well known that the extensor hallucis longus and anterior tibial muscle are more active during athletic involvement than the extensor digitorum longus muscles (2).

Group II. Traumatic Etiologies. Compartment syndromes following trauma may result in bleeding into a closed space secondary to fracture or soft tissue injury. The trauma causes bleeding and edema with increased pressure on the microcirculatory system resulting in ischemia. This also explains the reported cases of compartment syndromes following surgical procedures with closure of the fascial planes in the leg (11).

Group III. Vascular Injury, Disease or Thromboembolism Etiologies. In these cases major embarrassment to the circulation results in microcirculatory ischemia.

Lewis (9) pointed out that muscle ischemia is dependent upon microcirculation, not the major arterial and venous supply. The above etiologies, as pointed out by Bradley (2), suggest that in all cases there is microcirculatory embarrassment with resultant muscle ischemia.

Treatment

Initially, when one suspects a compartment syndrome, the patient should be put to bed rest, the limb elevated and ice packs applied. If edema and pain progress early, decompression of the involved compartment is mandatory. Early muscle damage occurs within 4 to 6 hr. and significant irreversible damage will be present at 18 hr. There is no place for watchful waiting in the management of this condition. Lueck and Ray (8) advocate complete fascial incision with split-thickness skin grafts in 5 to 7 days. They reported a case in which the anterior and posterior compartments were involved and two separate fascia incisions were required.

The author has noted two cases of severe shin splints (approaching early compartment syndromes), one in the anterior compartment and the other in the flexor compartment, which responded well to local injection of hyaluronidase. Following the intra-compartmental injections, the patients were placed on bed rest and ice packs and observed for any progression of pain and tension. Both patients were pain free within 4 hr. of treatment. A case of severe ischemic necrosis of the gastrocnemius and soleus muscle was noted in a patient who suffered from a drug overdose and spent the evening with extreme flexion compression being placed on the posterior superficial compartment, resulting in a posterior compartment syndrome with pressure necrosis of the gastrocnemius and soleus muscles.

Sequelae

The residual after effects of anterior compartment syndrome may be those of equinovarus with clawing of the toes and foot drop.

Summary

Compartment syndromes of the lower extremity have been presented with their etiologic factor appearing to be that of embarrassment of the microcirculation to the muscles. The microcirculation can be compromised secondary to strenous muscular activity with resultant edema and compression, direct trauma with resultant hemorrhage and compression, or major vascular disease with secondary microcirculatory effects. The importance of differentiating between the exercise idiopathic form of compartment syndrome and shin splints and strains was stressed. Patients with shin splints and strains respond readily to rest and the application of ice, whereas patients with compartment syndromes may progress to "woody tension" with extreme pain and loss of function as well as hypesthesia in the areas supplied by involved nerves. Loss of pulses secondary to compartment syndrome compression are a late finding and one should not wait for this sign before performing a surgical fasciotomy. Delay of treatment beyond 4 to 6 hr following onset may result in significant irreversible damage. It is hoped that early diagnosis and treatment, along with increased awareness, will lessen the disability following compartment syndromes in the lower extremity.

Appendix 1

References

1. Blandy, J. P. and Fuller, R.: March gangrene. J. Bone Joint Surg. 39B: 679, 1957.
2. Bradley, E. L.: The anterior tibial compartment syndrome. Surg. Gynecol. Obstet., 136: 298, 1973.
3. Craig, T. T.: *Comments in Sports Medicine*, p. 333, American Medical Association, Chicago, 1973.
4. Critchley, J. E.: The posterior tibial syndrome. Aust. N. Z. J. Surg., 42: 31, 1972.
5. Hughes, J. R.: Ischemic necrosis of the anterior tibial muscle due to fatigue. J. Bone Joint Surg., 30B: 581, 1948.
6. O'Donoghue, D. H.: *Treatment of Injuries to Athletes*, 2nd Ed., p. 601, W. B. Saunders, Philadelphia, 1970.
7. Willhoite, D. R. and Moll, J. H.: Early recognition and treatment of impending Volkmann's ischemia in the lower extremity. Arch. Surg., 100: 11, 1970.
8. Lueck, R. A. and Ray, R. D.: Volkmann's ischemia of the lower extremity. Surg. Clin. North Am., 52: 145, 1972.
9. Lewis, T.: *Vascular Disorders of the Limbs*, The Macmillan Co., London, 1936.
10. Carter, A. B., Richards, R. L. and Zachary, R. B.: Anterior tibial syndrome. Lancet, 2: 928, 1949.
11. Wollfort, G. F. G., Mogelvang, O. and Filtzer, H. S.: Anterior tibial compartment syndrome following muscle hernia repair. Arch. Surg., 106: 97, 1973.
12. French, E. Z. and Price, W. H.: Anterior tibial pain. Br. Med. J., 2: 1373, 1962.
13. Horn, C. P.: Acute ischemia of the anterior tibial muscle and the long extensors of the toes. J. Bone Joint Surg., 27A: 615, 1945.
14. Jones, D. A.: Volkmann's ischemia. Surg. Clin. North Am., 50: 329, 1970.
15. Spinner, M.: Importance of muscle variations as a factor in the deformity of Volkmann's contracture. Bull. Hosp. Joint Dis., 34: 48, 1973.
16. Weitz, E. M. and Carson, G.: The anterior tibial compartment syndrome in a 20 month old infant (a complication of the use of bow leg brace). Bull. Hosp. Joint Dis., 30: 16, 1969.
17. Coupland, G. A.: Anterior tibial syndrome following restoration of arterial flow. Aust. N. Z. J. Surg., 41: 338, 1972.
18. Dehne, E. and Kriz, F. K.: Slow arterial leak consequent to unrecognized arterial lacerations. J. Bone Joint Surg., 49: 372, 1967.
19. Jacob, J. E.: Vascular injuries in Viet Nam with special reference to compartment syndrome. Int. Surg., 57: 289, 1972.
20. Schonholtz, G. J.: Traumatic anterior tibial artery syndrome. South. Med. J., 65: 1343, 1972.
21. Benjamin, H. Z. and Nagler, W.: Peripheral nerve damage resulting from local hemorrhage and ischemia. Arch. Phys. Med. Rehabil., 54: 263, 1973.
22. Homes, W., Highet, W. B. and Seddon, H. J.: Ischemic nerve lesions occurring in Volkmann's contracture. Br. J. Surg., 32: 259, 1944.
23. Gardner, R. C.: Impending Volkmann's contracture following minor trauma to the palm of the hand. A theory of pathogenesis. Clin. Orthop., 72: 261, 1970.
24. Parkes, A.: Ischemic effects of external and internal pressure on the upper limb. Hand, 5: 105, 1973.
25. Scherr, D. D., Lichti, D. L. and Lambert, K. L.: Tissue viability assessment, with the Doppler Ultrasonic Flowmeter in acute injuries of extremities. J. Bone Joint Surg., 55A: 157, 1973.
26. Sheehan, G.: *Encyclopedia of athletic medicine*, p. 13, Runners World Magazine, California, 1972.
27. Eaton, R. G. and Green, W. Y.: Epimysiotomy and fasciotomy in the treatment of the Volkmann's ischemic contracture. Orthop. Clin. North Am., 3: 175, 1972.

Appendix 2

The Short Leg Syndrome

STEVEN I. SUBOTNICK, D.P.M., M.S.*

Asymmetries of limb length which cause lateral tipping of the pelvis and minor degrees of spinal curvature have been reported frequently in the literature.[2, 3, 5-10]

Pearson's progressive standing radiologic study of 830 school children from eight to thirteen years of age indicated that 93% had some degree of lateral asymmetry. Though compensation does occur, the structural asymmetry does not improve materially.[9] Klein demonstrated in 1953 that the greatest change in the development of lateral asymmetry occurs between the elementary and junior high school years, but the process continues into the senior high school ages.[5] Both Klein[6] and Fahey (special source of information) noted the relationship between foot pronation and lateral asymmetry.

Anderson stated that asymmetries of ¾ to 1½ inch require foot correction or a heel lift. Limb-length discrepancies of less than ¾ inch need no correction inasmuch as spontaneous compensation will take place.[1] However, the authors have found that limb-length discrepancies of ¼ inch or more, when associated with imbalance symptoms, do need correction. Limb-length discrepancies greater than ½ inch require that an adjustment layer of about half the thickness of the heel lift be added to the sole of the shoe to prevent equinus.[6] Deviations over 1½ inch may need a prosthetic device or, for severe discrepancies, surgery.

Limb-length discrepancies of the lower extremity often cause disabling problems for runners. Although major limb-length discrepancies are usually recognized at a young age, minor discrepancies are frequently unnoticed until symptoms ranging from low back pain to sciatica develop.[2 3 5 9] A careful examination of the patient may reveal asymmetry of the pelvis secondary to an anatomical or functional shortening of one limb. Pain in the low back, pelvis, hip or pain which radiates down the thigh (sciatica) can be secondary to other causes, including primary nerve disease or secondary nerve involvement.[1] A third cause is low backstrain which often accompanies asymmetry of the lower extremities. When examination has eliminated other causes of sciatica in the presence of limb-length discrepancies, heel lifts or orthoses can transform a runner with nagging, almost disabling pain into a pain-free athlete.

Types of Limb-Length Discrepancies

The basic measurement procedure for determining the symmetry or asymmetry of the posterior iliac spines is that recommended by

Lowman[8], Redler,[5] and Klein[6]. Lateral pelvic imbalance of ¼ inch or more was recorded, determined by the thickness of heel lift necessary to achieve balance of the pelvis (posterior iliac spine) and spinal column with the patient standing.

The patient should stand on a low table with feet slightly apart, legs parallel, knees straight ahead, arms hanging naturally to the sides. The investigator should palpate the posterior superior iliac spine. Calibrated blocks of 1/16 inch should be added until the pelvic spines are level. This measurement is basically for anatomical limb-length discrepancies. It fails to take into account the functional limb-length discrepancy secondary to unilateral excessive pronation of a foot.

The authors prefer to classify two types of limb-length discrepancies. The first is anatomical, in which there is an actual shortening of one limb, causing a tilt of the pelvis and a secondary compensation of the spinal column, resulting in scoliosis (Figures 1 and 2). The second is functional. It is secondary to abnormal positioning of the hip with muscle spasm or abnormal positioning of one foot causing abnormal pelvis rotation (Figure 3).

With structural limb-length discrepancy, both the anterior and posterior portion of the pelvis will usually be low on the side of the short leg. There may be a compensating curve of the spine convex to the short-leg side. The shoulder blade, scapula, on the long-limb side will drop and the arm on the long-leg side will appear longer than the arm on the short-leg side. If the scoliosis is secondary to the limb-length discrepancies, it will disappear when the patient is seated. If the limb-length discrepancy is secondary to scoliosis or a pelvic problem, it will persist while seated.

A flexible curvature of the spine may become less flexible and less rigid with the passing of time. The patient with the short-leg syndrome may compensate by externally rotating his foot and leg to provide for stability.[4] This complicates the problem because an externally rotated foot also has a valgus of the heel and associated collapse of the arch.[11] The external rotation of the leg on an internally-rotated femur causes the knee-joint to suffer. Klein commented on the relationship between externally-rotated legs and knee-joint pathology among athletes.[4]

If the patient has a functional limb-length discrepancy, the foot on the short-leg side will be externally rotated with the heel in valgus and the arch collapsed. The patient with the true limb-length discrepancy who compensates for lateral instability by externally rotating the foot has the same appearance. But when the patient with the functional discrepancy is examined, the rear pelvic spine will be higher on the short-leg side than on the long-leg side. Yet the front pelvic spine will be lower on the short-leg side than on the long-leg side. The internal rotation of the leg and thigh which accompanies pronation or flattening of the foot causes the pelvis to rotate asymmetrically, thus lowering the anterior pelvic spine and raising the posterior pelvic spine.

Differential Diagnosis of Limb-Leg Discrepancies

To examine for structural limb-length discrepancy, both heels should be placed in a perpendicular or neutral position, with the arches of both feet as close to normal as possible in normal gait angle.[11] The posterior pelvic spines should be palpated and differences in elevation noted. The anterior pelvic spines should likewise be palpated and noted. The compensation in a true limb-length discrepancy is ascertained by building up the heel of the short leg side, using different thicknesses of blocks, until the iliac spines are level. If the discrepancy is discovered in childhood or early adulthood, this compensating treatment may cause the curvature of the spine to disappear and improve the angle of gait.

For a functional limb-length discrepancy, both heels should be placed in neutral position, or close to vertical, with the arches of both feet normal. This will cause the anterior and posterior iliac spines to become level, the limb-length discrepancy to disappear and the curvature of the spine to straighten. The treatment for a functional limb-length discrepancy is therefore neutral arch control. This is accomplished by using orthotic devices made over a cast of the patient's foot while the foot is held in position of maximum function, the neutral position.

Occasionally, combinations of anatomic and functional limb-length discrepancies will occur and it may be necessary to prepare orthoses with a heel lift on the short-leg side.

At times, patient reactions are contrary to predictions. The patient's foot may function slightly pigeon-toed on the short-leg side, causing the arch of the foot to be elevated with external rotation of the leg as the foot is planted on the ground. The elevation of the arch may also cause some leveling of the pelvis.

Symptoms Accompanying Limb-Length Discrepancy

Symptoms accompanying limb-length discrepancies include sciatica and generalized low-back pain.[4,12] Pain in the hip joint and pain along the outside of one thigh or iliotibial band may accompany low back pain. Sciatica is a radiating nerve pain beginning in the low back and running down the inside of the thigh, sometimes to the inside of the foot. The pain is accentuated when the patient lies on his back and attempts a straight leg raise. The pain is also more severe when running uphill. Sciatic pain is often present on the short-leg side and may be associated with low back strain or herniation of an inter-vertebral disc.[12] Primary and secondary nerve involvement must be ruled out. When sciatica is secondary to limb-length discrepancy, the response to a heel lift or an orthosis is dramatic. Failure to obtain dramatic relief would indicate further consultation with other medical specialists.

Low back pain or back strain may be associated with sacroiliac joint involvement, a nagging pain over the buttocks. The patient would feel more comfortable seated and resting on the noninvolved buttocks. This pain likewise presents a formidable list of possible causes which should be investigated before the diagnosis of pain is deemed secondary to limb-length discrepancy.

FIGURE 1
Anatomical Short Leg

FIGURE 2
Functional Short Leg

FIGURE 3
Disappearance of Functional Short Leg With Orthotic Control

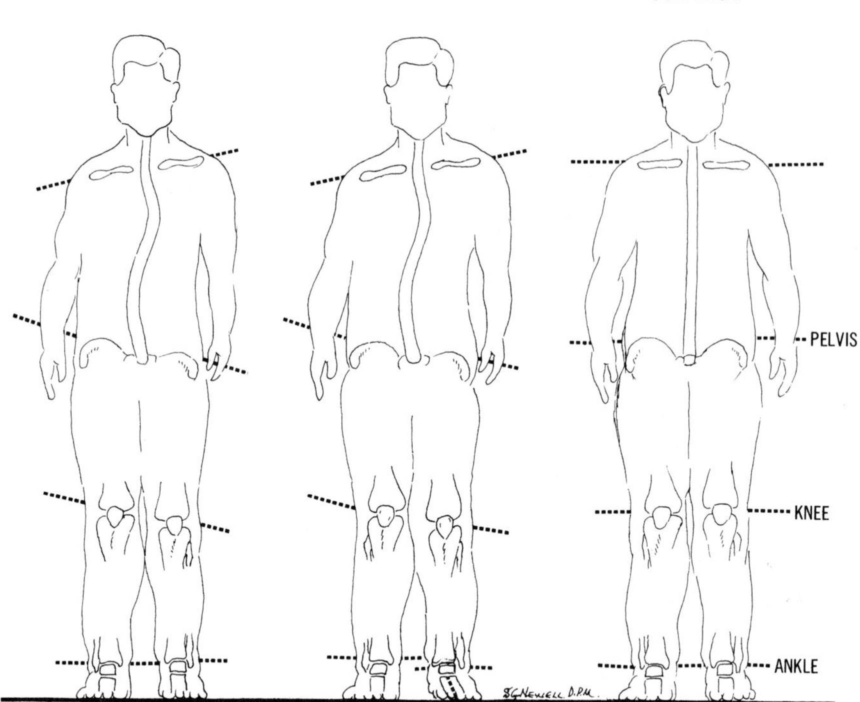

Summary

The importance of lower limb symmetry in the athlete was discussed. It was demonstrated that minor limb-length discrepancies which would cause little difficulty in the nonathlete can cause significant symptoms in the active athlete. The runner requires a symmetrical body frame. Symptoms secondary to structural or functional limb-length discrepancies frequently respond dramatically to heel lifts or to orthotic control of abnormal foot motion.

REFERENCES

[1] Anderson, W. V.: *Modern Trends in Orthopedics*, p. 1-22, Appleton-Century-Crofts, 1972.

[2] Beal, M. C.: Review of short leg problem. *J. Amer. Osteo. Assn.*, **50**:109-121, 1950.

[3] Green, W. T.: Discrepancy in leg length of lower extremities. *Am. Acad. Orthop. Surg., Instructional Course Lectures (VIII)*, J. W. Edwards Co., Ann Arbor, 1951.

[4] Klein, K. K.: Flexibility—strength and balance in athletics. *J. of N.A.T.A.*, **6**:62-65, 1971.

[5] Klein, K. K.: Progression of pelvic tilt in adolescent boys from elementary through high school. *Arch. of Phys. Med. Rehab.*, **54**:57-59, 1953.

[6] Klein, K. K. and Buckley, J. C.: Asymmetries of growth in pelvis and legs of growing children: summation of three-year study (1964-67). *Amer. Correct. Ther. J.*, **22**:53-55, 1968.

[7] Lovett, R. W.: *Lateral Curvature of Spine and Round Shoulders*, chapters 4, 7, 9, P. Blakiston's Son and Co., Philadelphia, 1912.

[8] Lowman, C. L. Colestock, C. and Cooper, H.: *Corrective Physical Education for Groups*, p. 63, A. S. Barnes, New York, 1937.

[9] Pearson, W. M.: Progressive structural study of school children, *J. Amer. Osteo. Assn.*, **51**:155-157, 1951.

[10] Redler, I.: Clinical significance of minor inequalities in leg length. *New Orleans Med. Surg. J.*, **104**:308-312, 1952.

[11] Sgarlato, T. E.: *A Compendium of Podiatric Biomechanics*, p. 60-65, C.C.P.M., San Francisco, 1971.

[12] Wiltse, L.: The effect of the common anomalies of the lumbar spine upon disc degeneration and low back pain. *Orthop. Clin.*, **2**:569-582, 1971.

SPECIAL SOURCES OF INFORMATION

[1] Fahey, J. F.: *Retarded leg syndrome* (mimeo.), Hollywood, California, 1971.

[2] Klein, K. K.: *Comparison of asymmetries in pelvis and legs of elementary and junior high school boys (1964-68)*. Dept. of Physical Education for Men, University of Texas at Austin, (mimeo), 1968.

Appendix 3

The Biomechanical Basis of Skiing

A Preliminary Report

STEVEN I. SUBOTNICK, D.P.M.*

Skiing is a series of closed kinetic chain rotations and movements which allow for the setting and unsetting of the ski edge to initiate and complete turns over varying surfaces (Figs. 1 and 2).

Biomechanic Basis of Skiing

Although skiing techniques vary, they all rely upon transverse rotations which result in closed chain pronation and supination to effect edge control.

The Austrian technique utilizes a preturn to release edges prior to a turn. The upper body transverse rotations accentuate transverse rotations of knee, legs and, finally, the skis.

The newer French method depends upon skier endurance and utilizes a thrust initiated at the knee joint. No matter which method is evaluated, one constant remains: transverse rotation of the limbs results in eversion or inversion of the skiis. The amount of eversion or inversion controls the ski edge setting.

Internal rotation results in closed chain pronation which results in eversion of the foot and ski (Figs. 1 and 10). A skier with his right ski downhill who turns into the hill would internally rotate his right lower extremity which would evert his right ski thus setting his right uphill edge. This allows the skier to "hold" the hill. The skier's left leg must externally rotate which inverts the left ski and sets the uphill edges of the uphill ski (Fig. 3).

Deformities Which Affect Skiing

It becomes apparent that deformities of the lower extremity which vary from the ideal perpendicular relationship between the leg and calcaneus (as a unit) and foot could affect a skier's ability to set edges.

The following deformities will be considered: tibial varum (Fig. 4), tibial valgum (Fig. 5), subtalar varus (Fig. 6) and forefoot varus (Fig. 7).

Tibial varum (Fig. 4) results in an increased outside ski edge. If more than 8 to 10 degrees of varus deformity is present it is virtually impossible to make a parallel turn without catching on the outside edge. Tibial varum is controlled by canting between the boot and the ski (Fig. 8).

---

* Assistant Professor of Biomechanics and Surgery, Director of First Year Residency Program, Co-Chairman of Biochemical Sports Podiatry Research Project, California College of Podiatric Medicine.

Figure 1. Effect of internal rotation.

Figure 2. Effect of external rotation.

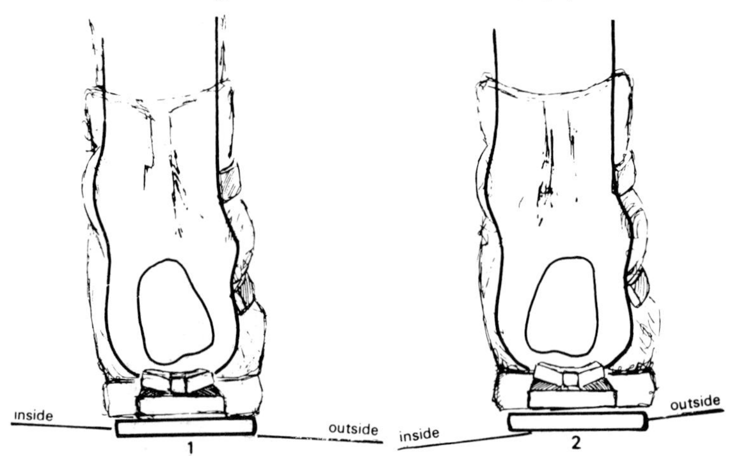

Figure 3. Effect of turning into a hill.

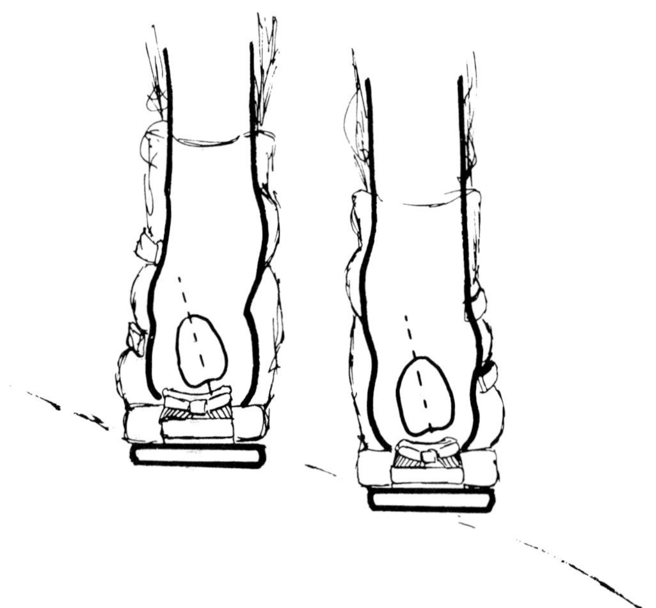

Tibial valgum places more stress upon the inside edge which will result in difficult uphill edge control and edge catching on the flats. It is controlled by cants between the boot and ski (Fig. 9).

Subtalar varum when held in a firm ski boot will present with the same effects as tibial varum. Because this is a deformity within the foot it is controlled by a device within the boot. A subtalar varum which compensates within a loose or soft boot decreases the total pronatory motion available

Figure 4. Tibial varum. Figure 5. Tibial valgum. Figure 6. Subtalar varus.

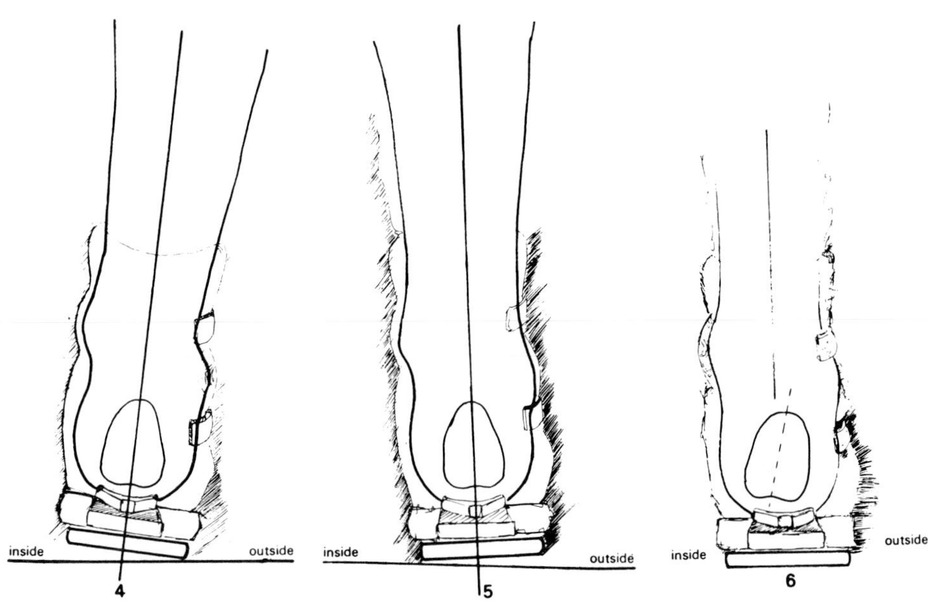

Figure 7. Forefoot varus and compensation.

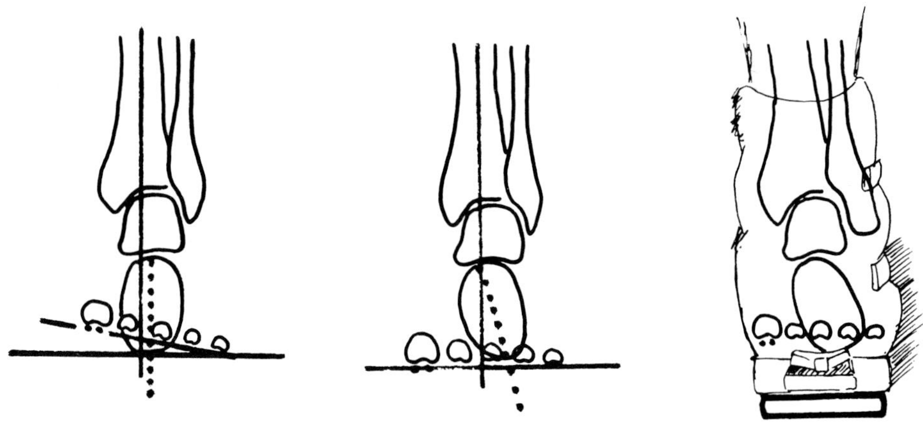

and results in poor edge control as well as contorted positions in an attempt to set a downhill edge (Fig. 10).

Forefoot varus (Fig. 7) will cause similar effects as a compensated subtalar joint varus. The boot must evert which reduces pronatory motion available. Full control is maintained with in-the-boot orthotics.

Any of the skeletal deformities discussed, or combination of them, can result in compensation as seen in Figures 11 and 12.

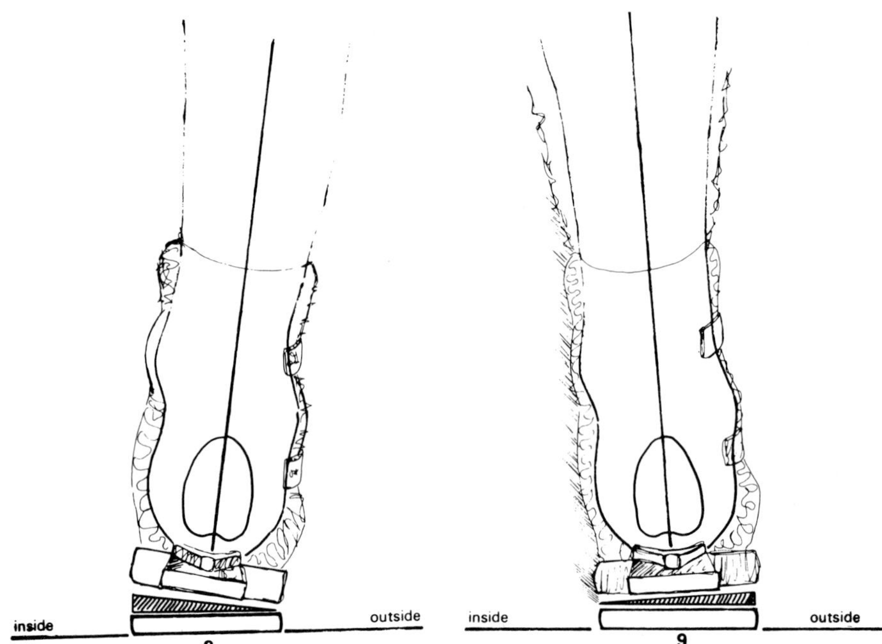

Figure 8. Tibial varum and cant.

Figure 9. Tibial valgum and cant.

Skiing Compensations

In an original article by Warren Witherel, who is the Director of Alpine Training Centers, Burke Mountain, entitled: "If You Can't Ski Parallel, Cant," appearing in *Skiing*, January 1971 issue, over 1000 racers and recreational skiers were tested. Four out of five were not able to stand perfectly flat on the soles of their skiis in the straight running position of skiing. Instead, they rode their outside edges.

Skiers who ride their outside edges have a great deal of difficulty parallel skiing, and end up stemming or hopping as they begin their turns. They are prone to catching uphill or outside edges.

It is estimated that 80% of the population has some lower extremity or foot abnormality causing symptoms from the moderate complaints of postural fatigue to the more severe complaints of rearfoot and forefoot pain secondary to abnormal biomechanical forces. Mr. Witherel's research appears to support this data.

Normally, the skier who rides the outside edges of his skis flattens out his foot to compensate for a varus deformity. This allows for a flat ski. Since ski boots increase in stiffness as they increase in expense, the more expensive boots, for the more advanced skiiers, disallow motion within the foot. Disallowing motion within the foot disallows the normal compensatory subtalar joint pronation.

This forces the skier to contort his body position to ski parallel. Witness the skier who tucks his downhill ski leg into the space behind his uphill knee, thus internally rotating his downhill leg to set the inside edge (Fig. 12).

Skiers will best compensate for varus deformities in their lower extremities by stemming, hopping, tucking in their downhill knee, or a combination of the above and some other contorting maneuvers. This is at the expense of comfortable skiing, and leads to postural symptoms, as well as injuries from catching uphill ski edges. A more satisfactory solution would be to place a cant between the boot and the ski to allow even distribution of weight through a flat ski while the subtalar joint is in a neutral position. This allows the skis to lie perfectly flat against the snow when a straight running position is assumed. This also allows the ski edges to be equally edged when transversing or turning without any contorsion on the part of the skier. Tibial and leg deformities require a cant. Rearfoot and forefoot deformities require an orthotic to be worn in the boot. The orthotic is fabricated from a neutral foot cast (Figs. 10 and 13).

Canting

When Needed. Mr. Witherel explains that there are seven clues to indicate when one may require a cant.

Figure 10. Compensation for varus subtalar joint with internal rotation.

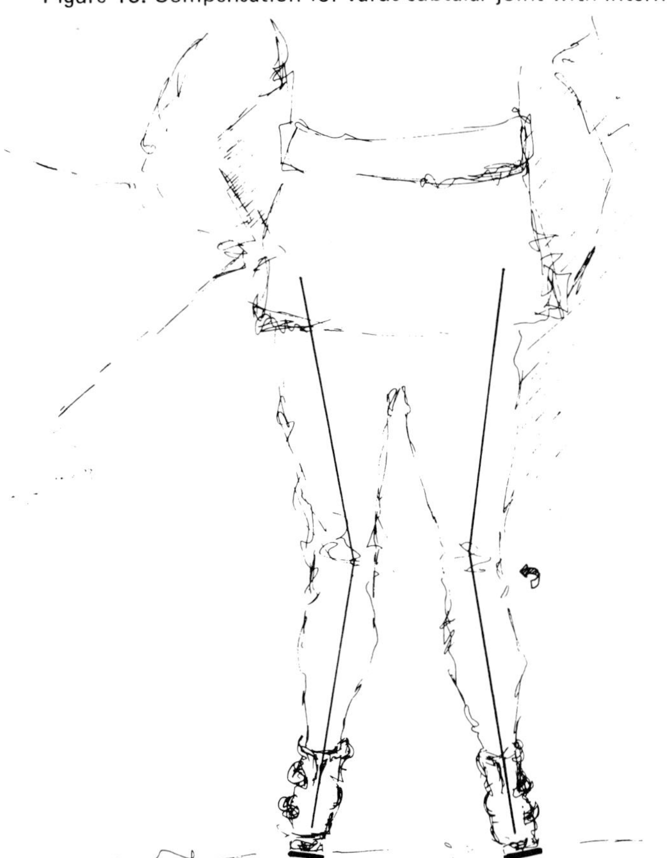

Fiaure 11. Turning with downhill knee tucked and behind.

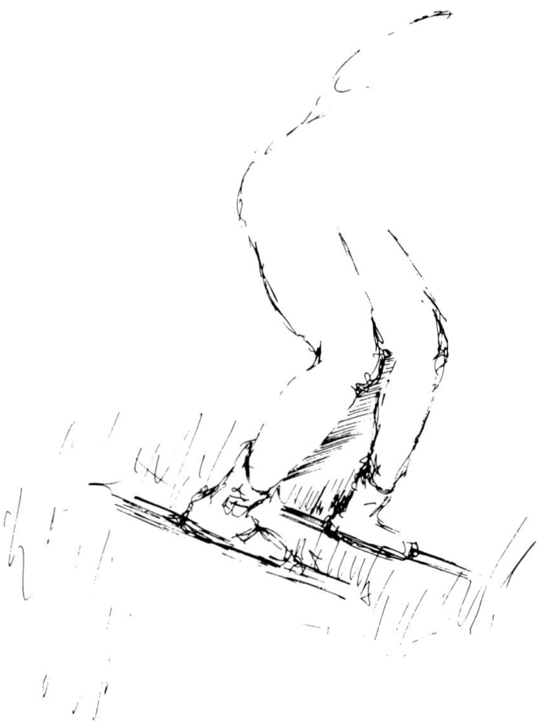

Figure 12. Turning with downhill knee tucked and behind, and the effect on the edges.

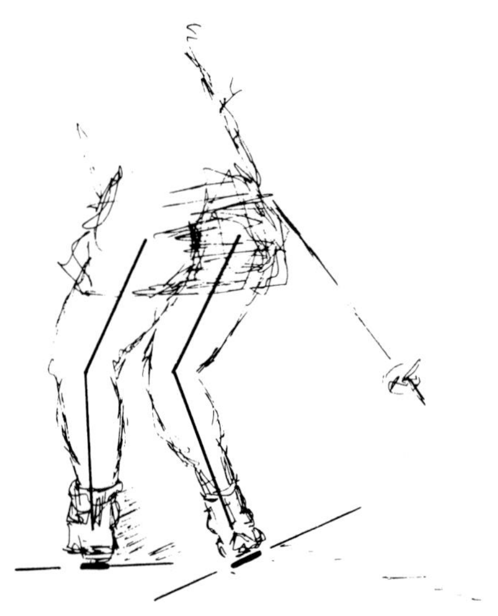

Figure 13. Controlled forefoot varus with "in-shoe" post.

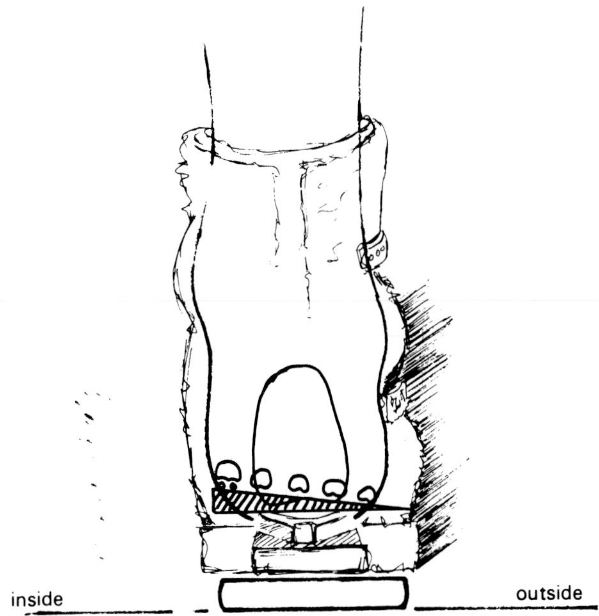

1. When you wear down the outside edges of the heels of your shoes

2. When you're standing across the hill in a transverse position, if you can't equally edge your uphill and downhill skis and if, to compensate for this, you have to tuck in your downhill knee

3. If you can't break the stemming habit, no matter how many lessons you have had. Mr. Witherel notes that if you need more than 8 to 10 degrees of a cant, it is virtually impossible to make a parallel turn without catching your outside edge.

4. If you have to hop to initiate a turn

5. If you lean to the inside of your turn, or depend too much on your outside ski

6. If, despite excellent skis, you have a great deal of difficulty holding on a side hill on ice

7. If you turn in one direction better than in another direction.

How Much Needed. Although it is possible to cant by trial and error, it is safer to have a measurement by an expert prior to canting (Fig. 14) and to follow the rule that undercanting is better than overcanting. You must be measured with your ski boot both on and off, your knees must be flexed into a normal skiing position with the boots buckled to normal tightness and you must be standing on a firm surface. The amount of motion in the boot can then be evaluated. With the neutral position first evaluated without the boot, the booted lower extremity is placed neutral. The actual varus deformity in the lower one third of the leg is then measured. The degree of the deformity corresponds to the degree of the cant. Subtalar or forefoot deformity requires boot control and is measured by the standard podiatric biomechanical principals.

Where to Cant. Preliminary evaluation of where to cant has revealed that for a problem within the leg itself, such as tibial varum, the canting should be between the boot and the ski and the cant should be long enough to go underneath the bindings.

Mr. Witherel has observed that, inside the boot, control is useful for correcting the effects of flat feet or weak arches which produce conditions very similar to that of a bow-legged skier with normal arches. These are the rearfoot and forefoot varus conditions of this report.

Commercial products like the newer ski boots which have cants built within them are, for good reasons, not custom-built and usually not canted enough for a skier with a moderate to severe deformity in his lower extremity. Likewise, the full-length cant insoles commercially available are usually not canted sufficiently. If they are canted sufficiently, they are of limited use because the boots become too tight on the raised aspect of the insole.

Discussion of Boots

For skiers with rearfoot or forefoot deformities the ideal would be to have a neutral orthotic fabricated, then place the orthotic and foot in a boot shell

Figure 14. Measurement of tibial varum for cant.

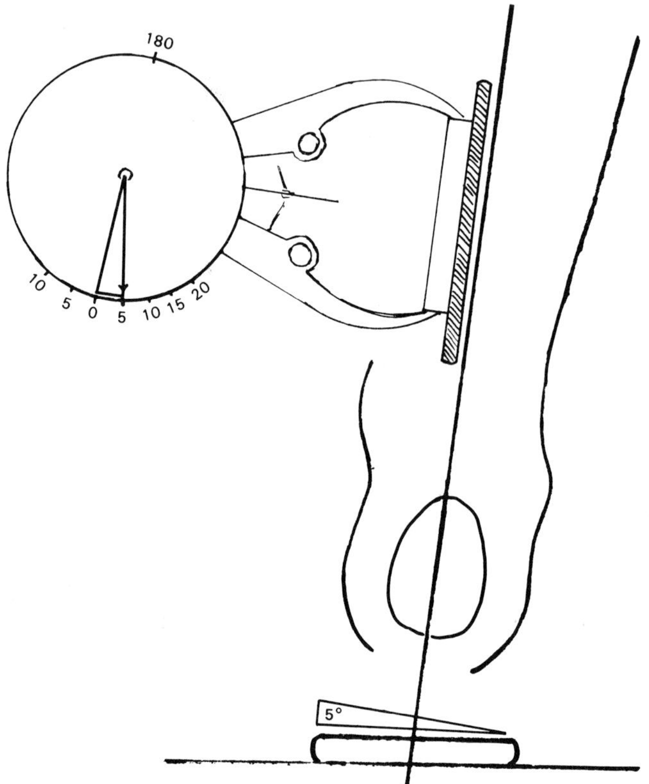

with weightbearing and foam inject. The skier would thus utilize the orthotic when skiing. For non-foam boots enough boot clearance must be available to allow for an orthotic.

Foot pressure points such as the first and fifth metatarsal heads and malleoli (ankle bones) must be accommodated. Attention should also be focused on anterior ankle friction and abrasions secondary to the forward cant in competition boots.

Boot manufacturers as well as binding manufacturers should be aware of canting requirements for tibial varum so that boot soles as well as bindings will function well with cants. A boot which allows for frontal plane adjustment seems practical as long as neutral lower extremity positions are appreciated.

Results of Canting Tests

Twenty-five skiers, including students from the California College of Podiatric Medicine and the author, were given biomechanical evaluations and orthotics were constructed accordingly to be worn inside of ski boots. Skiers with forefoot deformities were balanced with Rohadur® orthotics made from a neutral cast. Rearfoot deformities were compensated for by posting between boot and ski utilizing cants.

Moving pictures were taken in slow motion with and without cant devices and showed that, with canting and control in the boot, there was less tendency for the uphill ski to lag behind at the beginning of the turn.

After a 2-year trial period, results indicate that in most cases improvement in skiing technique was noted, especially with improved ability to control ski edges. In short, parallel skiing was accomplished with greater ease. Two of the skiers had equinus deformities to such an extent that even pronated orthotics were not tolerated well and they were considered failures.

Further research will include continued use of slow motion films of skiers with differing skiing abilities before and after control. It is expected that skiing will be made more enjoyable and safer with proper biomechanical evaluation of the lower extremities, canting and boot control.

Author's Note

Caution should be exercised initially when using orthotics and cants, as there is a tendency to over-edge. My personal experience indicates that I am able to ski on a flatter edge with less exertion.

Acknowledgments. I would like to acknowledge gratefully the following persons for their assistance with this project: T. E. Sgarlato, D. P. M., Director of Biomechanics and Professor of Surgery; Mr. John Ruch, a senior student for drawing the illustrations for this paper; Ms. Reggie L. Steele and Ms. Thelma R. Valentino, typists; and Anglo-Scandinavian Corporation, Burlingame, Calif., for donation of ski boots and bindings.